NUMBER 238

THE ENGLISH EXPERIENCE

ITS RECORD IN EARLY PRINTED BOOKS
PUBLISHED IN FACSIMILE

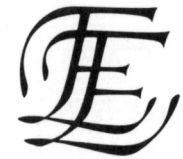

WILLIAM CLOWES

TREATISE
FOR THE ARTIFICIALL CURE
OF STRUMA

LONDON 1602

DA CAPO PRESS
THEATRVM ORBIS TERRARVM LTD.
AMSTERDAM 1970 NEW YORK

The publishers acknowledge their gratitude
to the Syndics of Cambridge University Library
for their permission to reproduce
the Library's copy
(Shelfmark: K.16.33.)

S.T.C. No. **5446**
Collation: A-K^4

Published in 1970 by
Theatrum Orbis Terrarum Ltd.,
O.Z. Voorburgwal 85, Amsterdam

&

Da Capo Press
- a division of Plenum Publishing Corporation -
227 West 17th Street, New York, 10011
Printed in the Netherlands
ISBN 90 221 0238 6

A RIGHT FRVTEFVLL AND APPROOVED

Treatise, for the Artificiall Cure of that Malady called in Latin *Struma*, and in English, the *Evill*, cured by Kinges and Queenes of England.

Very necessary for all young Practizers of Chyrurgery.

Written by WILLIAM CLOWES, one of her Maiesties Chyrurgions, in the yeare of our Lord. 1602.

Imprinted at London by Edward Allde. 1602.

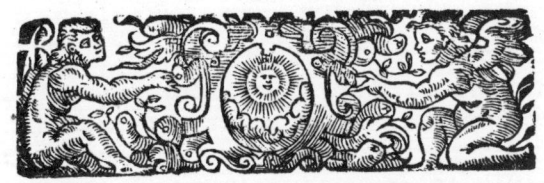

The Epistle to the Reader.

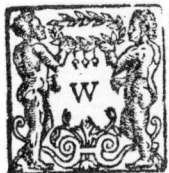Hen I considered with my selfe (curteous and friendly Reader)the graue & wise saying of Tully: that Honour maintaineth Artes, wherby men are greatly addicted to study: So, as it is said, if a man looke into the course of this world, and into humaine affayres, yee shall finde that such Artes as serue the peoples necessity,& haue their necessarie vse in the common wealth, haue been greatly esteemed, and the Professors thereof highly rewarded. Amongst a number of which lawdable Artes & Sciences, let vs make our consideration of Chirurgery, the maintainer and restorer of our healthes: For it is a most true receiued opinion amongst worthy writers, that Chirurgery is (indeede) an ancient part of Phisicke, as it appeareth by Iaques Guillemeau of Orleans ordinary Chirurgian to the now French King: who auoucheth, that before Phisick was inuented, created, or found out, Chirurgery was practized, and sufficiently knowne in al places: as it appeareth (saith he) by the testimonie of Homer, in the second booke of his Ilyades: who wrote the valiant enterprises, and trauels of Vlisses, as did Titus Liuius, the worthy actes and monuments of the Ancient Romaines. Moreouer, it is said, that Apollo for his skill, and Æsculapius his sonne, were honoured (as Gods) of al the worthy Grecians; Podalerius and Machaon the two sonnes of Æsculapius, were had in great honour & reputation, at the siedge of Troy, vnder Agamēnon, Captaine of the Grecians. Moreouer, Hippocrates the paragon of all ages, was highly esteemed by the Athenians: Erasistratus, of Noble Saleucus: Diocles, of Antigonus: Oribasius, of Iulian: Dioscorides, of Marcus Antonius, and Cleopatra: who followed the warres ouer Ægipt, Parthia, Armenia, Persia, India and Siria: and all to augment and encrease their knowledge & skill. Last of all the said Worthyes, I heere nominate Gallen, who is called the light of all good learning : and hee also was greatly honoured of Traian the Emperour, and he followed the warres with

A 2   him,

Epistle to the Reader.

him, ouer all Asia and Europa: I had heere likewise thought good to haue spoken somewhat of Paracelsus, but I must confesse his Doctrine hath a more pregnant sence, then my wit or reach is able to construe: onely this I can say by experience, that I haue practised certaine of his inuentions Chirurgicall, the which I haue found to be singular good, & worthy of great commendations. How be it, much strife I know there is betwen the Galenistes and the Paracelsians, as was in times past betweene Aiax and Vlisses, for Achilles Armour. Notwithstanding, for my part I will heere set vp my rest & contentation, how impertinent and vnseemely so euer it make shew: That is to say, if I finde (eyther by reason or experience) any thing that may be to the good of the Patients, and better increase of my knowledge & skil in the Arte of Chirurgery, be it eyther in Galen or Paracelsus; yea, Turke, Iewe, or any other Infidell: I will not refuse it, but be thankefull to God for the same. How be it, I will in no wise meddle with their Infidelity, though I imbrace their knowledge and skill in humane veritves and inuentions, be it eyther in Phisicke or Chirurgery, or any of the other laudable Sciences. Now I will discourse no further, vntill a more fit opportunity be offered: But very briefly I meane heere to demonstrate and deliuer vnto the friendly Reader, the cure of a certaine vnnaturall tumor or abscesse, called in Latin, Struma: of the Arabians, Steophala: but generally, in English, it is called, the Kings or Queenes Euill: A disease repugnant to nature: which grieuous malady is knowne to be miraculously cured & healed, by the sacred hands of the Queenes most Royall Maiesty, euen by Diuine inspiration and wonderfull worke and power of God, aboue mans skill, Arte and expectation: Through whose Princely Clemency, a mighty number of her Maiestyes most Loyall subiects, and also many strangers borne, are dayly cured and healed, which otherwise would most miserably haue perished. For many of them (their pouerty was such) were not able to pay but a very little or nothing at all for their cure. And so I heere conclude, that as God by his diuine giftes, doth cure this Strumous Malady: so also of his great goodnes, he doth giue Artificiall giftes, for the curing of the said Infirmity. But whereas Artificiall giftes doe many times fayle thee, doe his deuine giftes take place & reuaile: as after more at large shall appeare.

William Clowes, one of her Maiesties Chirurgions.

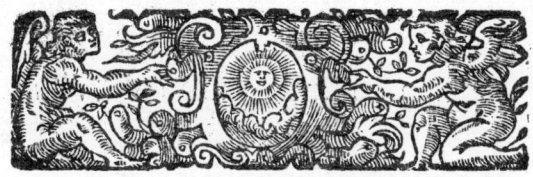

Tho: Bonhami, in Medic: Doct.
Exastichon: In laudem Authoris.

CLVSIVS es dictus, meliús sed APERTIVS esses:
    Clausa aperîs, alios quæ latuêre prius,
Regalisq́ mali causam, auxiliúq́ RECLVDENS,
    Doctus Apollineæ porrigis artis opem.
Multi Asclepiadæ frustra hanc petiêre coronam,
    Solus habê, palmam hanc tradit Apollo tibi.

FINIS.

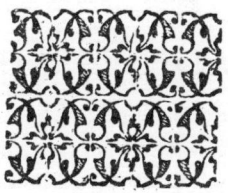

Thomas Folkys of Lincolns Inne
Gent. in commendation of William
Clowes his booke.

BY long experience and by practiſe great,
Time hath affoorded to this painfull man
A helpfull cure, which heeretofore to treate,
The greateſt Clarkes haue doubted how & whan.
To cure the ſame giue *Clowes* due praiſe therefore,
That hath performed this and many more.

But yet conceiue, this is not *Clowes* his cure,
Our Soueraigne Lady, and his Miſtris Queene:
Seemes well content her man may put in vre
So much as ſhe affoordes; as may be ſeene
By *Clowes* his ſcope, the reſt ſhe challengeth,
As Queene annoynted and by Royall birth.

Then Phiſicke yeeld; giue place Chirurgery;
The Rationall and Practicke for this paine
Are both a like: her Peereleſſe Maieſtie
Healeth by God alone, Arte is but vaine.
This ſhe performes, to write I muſt ſurceſſe,
Her hidden skill no pen can well expreſſe.

How much then are we to the high God bound,
For ſending vs this Princeſſe heere on earth?
Within whoſe breſt, ſuch helpes are dayly found,
As heales her ſubiectes at the point of death.
She cures, ſhe cares, ſhe ſaues vs all by skill:
She hurteth none, but helpes with louing will.

Liue, liue for aye: what humour leadeth me?
I gan to write in *VVilliam Clowes* his praiſe;
Her onely name hath drawne my quill I ſee.
And daunted ſo my ſence by ſundry waies:
That like as *Zenxis* ſhaddowed his intent,
With ſome conceipt, ſo I the ſame way went.

FINIS.

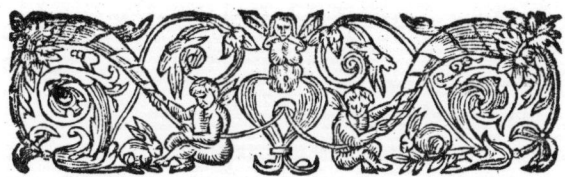

Thomas Parkin Chyrurgie professor.

THe happy sacred hand, of our dread Soueraigne Queen,
  The Princely louing zeale, of her most Royall heart,
  Throughout her highnes land, her subiects al haue seen
To cure, to helpe, to heale, our care, our harme, our smart.
  To God all glory for her Gratious Raigne,
  To her all blessings, that on earth remaine.

And thankes, and thankes to *Clowes*, for this his zealous toyle,
In searching out the light, of *Chyrons* hidden skill:
And for the loue he shewes, to Countryes natiue soyle,
To practise, finde, and write, for all instructions still,
  Let *Clowes* be loued his fame and him defend,
  Who, what he prooued, the same for vs hath pend.

FINIS.

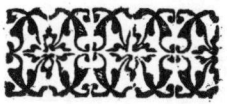

Iosua Smarlet practitioner of *Phisicke* and Chyrurgery.

LET him giue thankes, that hath not else
    wherewith to gratifie
  His friend, that giues so great a gift
    to cure the *Strumacye*.
Nor that alone he comprehends,
    his helpfull remedyes:
Dissolue hard *Tumors*, colde *Inflations*,
    Fluxes and *Nodosities*:
Approaching age makes wisdome in his tongue,
  His heart gain'd Arte, when yet his yeeres were young.

He *Chimicke* Arte disclaimes to know,
    yet *Ladanum* he showes:
And many good collections more,
    (his pen doth heere disclose)
The quintessence of his whole life,
    in gayning skyll consumed:
He graunteth franckly to thine vse,
    with Science sweets perfumed.
Future times shall praise his meditation,
  And him repose in Heauens consolation.

Base ignoraunce bids me conceale,
    mine owne vnworthynes:
True loue to Arte compelles me more,
    T'eschewe vngratefulnes.
Impute my faults t'affection's force,
    and his well deseruing,
That spends his sprites and restlesse houres,
    in mans life preseruing.
The long experience and good Arte of this our *Clowes*,
  Deserueth rightly more reward then Lawrell bowes.

FINIS.

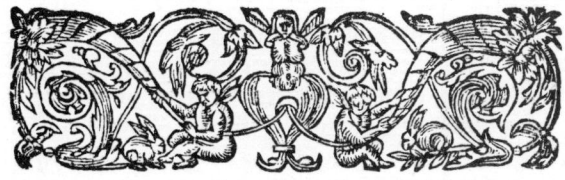

AN INTRODUCTION,

With an Apologie or answere to certaine malicious back-byters.

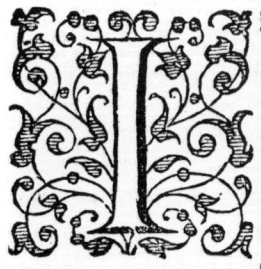T is certainly affirmed, and confidently reputed and holden, of diuers worthy Phisitians and Chirurgians, both Ancient and such as haue florished of late yéeres, which haue intreated of the Cure of the before named dolorous Maladie: and they all by one vniforme consent and voice, conclude and agrée, that it is a Glandulus Tumour or swelling, hard, knotty, and kyrnelly, hauing their beginning and growing, contrarie and besides nature, and is ingendred of grosse matter and Phlegme: And (as saith Iacobus Ruffus) they are most commonly included within their peculiar Cistis, filme or skinne, as is Steatoma, Atheroma, and Meliceris: which aforesaid skin is knowne to be engendred of a colde congealed, tough, glewish humour or substance of the Kirnels, whereof a skinne is made which compasseth them about: Howbeit I haue séene (and also it is a most experimented truth) that some kindes of these Phlegmaticall Abscessions,

B   when

when they haue béen besiedged as it were, or beset with vehement daungerous accidents, as héereafter shall be declared, which in continuance of time haue bin ẏ cause they haue growne corrupted & vnmoueable, or fixed vnto the parts adioyning: whereby after there hath bin seperation made, there hath not bin found any bladder or skin at all, notwithstanding the great care & diligence that then was had.

This most miserable infirmity (saith Paulus Ægineta) doth scituate or seate it self in the fore part of ẏ necke & vnder the Chin: also on the sides of the chéekes, & sometime spreadeth it selfe vpon the brest, & vnder the Armepits, & Groynes, & some be déeply lodged a far off in the flesh, & also do oftentimes possesse the great Vaines and Arteryes called Carotides: And those that are thus vered & subiect to this troublesome Infirmity, are for the most part Phlegmatick persons, greatly giuen to ouermuch Idlenes & slouthfulnes of life, & are addicted to excessiue and inordinate eating of grosse & Flegmaticke meates: which manifolde Malady, I haue also found by experience, that the Cure thereof stretcheth it selfe beyond the bounds of other ordinary sicknesses & diseases. Cornelius Celsus likewise saith, that Scrophula is a Tumour, in the which are certaine kyrnels ingendred of matter and bloud, and doe most chiefly grow in the fore part of the Necke, & in the Arme-pits, the Groyne, & in the sides, and hath bin found in Womens brestes.

Vigo a man (for his learning and experience in this Cure, & in many other great Infirmities) as it appeareth, was wonderfully graced with the good opinion and fauour of the time wherein hee liued, & since his death greatly honoured by dyuers learned Writers, and many other men famous in Phisicke and Chyrurgery: He also sayth, that Scrophula taketh the name of Scropha, which signifieth a Sow, that is a Gluttonous

of the *Struma*.

tious and Phlegmaticke beaste: and it groweth in them by reason of their ouermuch eating. There be other some againe which say, that it is called Scrophula, eyther because that Sowes which giue sucke be subiect to this disease, and that is by reason of their greedy eating: or else because the Sow that giueth Milke brings foorth many young ones at once.

Now heere it is to be further noted, that Vigo doth not promise or warrant alwaies, and to euery one a certaine absolute Cure, but doth (as I, and many other also haue done) ascribe the praise and dignity therof vnto Kings and Queenes of England, and of France: In deede I haue oftentimes read, and I haue also been credibly enformed by Maister Francis Rasis, and Maister Peter Lowe, two of the French Kinges Chyrurgians, that the French King doth also Cure many Strumous people, onely by laying on of his hand, and saying: God make thee whole, the King toucheth thee; or, The King toucheth thee, the Lord make thee whole.

It is further said, that this disease happeneth not alwayes vnto young children, which bee subiect to much crudity, & rawe humours by voracity: but likewise vnto middle aged persons, of a stronger constitution; and also vnto very olde folkes. Many therefore imitating Vigo and other of our Sages, & graue learned Forefathers, doe affirme that these Scrophulous Tumours bee the lesse daungerous to be cured by the Arte of Chyrurgery, which is taken in the beginning of the sicknes, so far foorth as it wil please Almighty God to giue a grace and blessing to our labours. But vndoubtedly, if it be of any long continuance, the Cure thereof may proue very hard and difficult: yea, if it be in the bodies of yong persons: But in olde folkes I haue obserued very sildome, that they do receiue any curatiō perfectly,

Hip: Aphor. sect.3.

B 2 by

by the Arte of Chirurgery. I meane, that it is then aboue my learning and weake capacity to cure the same, if the disease bee confirmed, hauing certaine occult and hidden, hard, knotty, kyrnelly swellings, (being deepely lodged and placed in the flesh) but especially about Trachea Arteria, or the winde Pipe, or neer the Nerui Recurrentes, or amongst the great Veynes and Arteries before named: these (indeede) I holde to bee for the most part very daungerous to be attempted, for feare of violating or touching the said principall Vessels, eyther by incision or Caustick remedies, which often times bring with them many vnfortunate Symptomes or iniurious accidents, as heereafter more at large shall appeare.

Also, it is hard to cure a noysome, corrupt and malignant vlcerous Struma, which doth many times degenerate into incurable, Cancerous & rebellious Phistulous Vlcers: Likewise, I hold it for a certaine truth, that the Cure is not to be attempted by the Arte of Chirurgery, if a man haue it by inheritance, and so naturally borne from their Parents: These kindes of Scropholus abcessions doe rather presage a Diuine and holy curation, which is most admirable to the world, that I haue seene and knowne performed and done by the sacred and blessed hands of the Queenes most Royall Maiesty, whose happinesse and felicity the Lord long continue.

But sith the barrennesse of my learning, and wit is such, and that my memorie will not affoord mee, heere orderlie to set downe in fewe words, that which I doe conceiue and vnderstand, touching this my determined purpose, for the Cure of this haynous Maladie: which, in the Pilgrimage of my practize and contemplations, I haue most diligentlie obserued, not onely by mine owne selfe, with such portion of knowledge as the Lord

hath

of the *Struma*.

hath endued me withall: But also I haue béen a diligent and a painfull obseruer of the labours and practises of others, being men of great knowledge and sound iudgement in the Arte: Wherefore to make héere manifest, the cause which hath pricked mee héere forward to leaue my other affaires, and so to drawe me from my ordinarie practises and studies, being more beneficiall for my maintenances, is not that I goe about héereby to impaire the credit or reputation of others, being more aunccient Professors. It is (the Lord God knoweth) farre from my true meaning, they are those whome I loue, honour and reuerence: Neyther doe I héer ambitiously goe about with the swéet impression of fayre promises (greater then my abilitie is) to teach and instruct, or curiously to set downe, a better and perfecter way of curing this haynous Malady (then others more learned men before me) I may not well say so. Neuerthelesse, he hardlie may be accompted for a good Souldier, which hath learned no more then his Captaine hath taught him: or a barren sconce, that hath no inuentions in it: But I will confesse héere the onely cause, (why I haue enterprized, or taken vpon me to write of this forenamed Infirmitie) is I protest, a token of my loue and diligence towards all young Practisers of this noble Arte of Chirurgerie, (howsoeuer otherwise, a painfull and tedious trauel vnto me.) Notwithstanding, I could in no wise satisfie the expectation of certaine of my vnfained friends, but that I must make here a true & briefe rehearsall of my owne obseruations and knowledge, touching the cure of the foresaid Euill, which a long time I haue practised. How be it, being sorry to minister offence to any, by reason of publication héereof. Notwithstanding, I haue béen crediblie enformed, and also it is vnto my selfe well knowne, there bee some whome I litle suspected, and lesse thought vpon, would

An Apology to answere certaine reproachfull back-biters.

B 3 haue

haue béen so wilfully bent, without iust cause to giue occasion of offence, and did séeme as it were to repine and mislike of this my enterprise: and as it were, did partly reiect my knowledge and iudgement, concerning the Cure before named: and in the presence of certaine persons of good sort, brake out with ambitious curiosity, and said I was not capable of the Theoricke of this my Subiect, and so wanted knowledge of my selfe to publish these matters, which I haue héere taken vpon mee in some measure to performe: and thus went about, not onely to discredit mee, but likewise to put me to vtter silence, as though I had spent all the daies of my life in the rude woodes or wilde Forrest of Ignorance. Which thing as it gréeued me to heare, so in maner it forced mee to answere: Let these men sooth themselues (I say) neuer so much, they are knowne to be of no such déep learning nor exquisite Literature, as they would make the world beléeue: Howbeit, if it please these enuious men to speake & iudge of me with equity & right: it is wel knowne to most men, that I haue studied & practised this worthy Arte of Chirurgery, sithence the 4. yeare of her Maiesties Raigne, Anno Dom. 1563. Where, first I serued in her Highnes wars at New-hauen, vnder the commaund of the Right Honorable Ambrose Earle of Warwicke, Knight of the Noble Order of the Garter, then Lieuetenant of the Army & Forces in those parts. After w̄ seruice being ended & before, I was appointed Chirurgian, to serue in her Maiesties Nauy in her ships Royall, & also in other men of war: within a smal time after, I was imployed in the Hospitalles in London, and there practised the said Arte of Chirurgery for certaine yéeres, vntill I was sent for vnto the wars in the Low Countries, by ẏ Noble Earle of Leicester: and further, commaunded by her Maiesty, with all spéed to repaire vnto the said Earle,

He that will vse Chyrurgery must needly follow the wars & attend on forraine Armies. Hipo. Lib. de Medic.

where

Where I continued for the space of 9. Moneths: & since & before I haue had conference, & also often practised, with the best and skilfullest Chyrurgians, both English and Strangers, within the City of London and else where: and now as it were, partly ouer-worne with yeares and Seruices. Notwithstanding, by her Maiesties fauour and good liking (whome the Almighty long preserue) now I am sworne & admitted one of her Highnes Chirurgians. And therefore in all reasonable likely-hood, I am not so barren or grosse witted, and vnlearned in the Arts, as some haue termed mee to bee. And yee shall further vnderstand, it was not long before, it pleased some of them to say, they had graced me with the good opinion they had of me: and moreouer stood in the gap of my defence against other such, which then were also sore troubled with the Fixe of a fowle mouth, & vsed me at their pleasures for their common Tabletalke, with scoffing, fleering, and deriding aboue manners and modesty. The same being tolde mee, me thought it was a strange alteration: howbeit, I did take their good spæches very kindly, and so would haue done still, if it had pleased them to continue in the same good opinion of me, or to haue bin silent. But it is truly said, Hanibal knew wel how to subdue the Romanes, yet he knew not how to entertaine his Victories. It is not enough for a man to haue begun a good worke, vnlesse he stil preseuer & continue in the same: Wherfore I wil heere abreuiate my spæches, wishing to God, that this my labor were so perfect, that I næded not to regard the curious examination & censure of any aduersary: neyther will I detaine you with many moe circumstances, but here acknowledge my own vnworthynes. And therfore I besæch thæ friendly Reader, in a word to suffer mee with pacience to signifie vnto you, that I doe not hære peremptorily goe about to teach or instruct

He that pitch doth touch, shall defiled be with such

such

such persons which are already grounded in the principles and knowledge of this Arte: But my onely meaning is to direct my whole course, according (as I haue obserued) the best learned haue hæretofore done in all times and ages, that is vnto the Iunior or yonger Chirurgions: who, as it were, haue made but an entrance into the practice of the said facultie, whose skill (peraduenture) is as yet not so profound, that they are able to search or obtaine ỹ knowledge out of strange tongues, so farre fourth that they cannot possibly in a short time come to the highest of that knowledge, which they hartely wish for. Indæde, it is (I suppose) vnpossible in the whole course of mans life, euen vnto that Period, which (of the Learned) is called Mans Age: that hee is able without great care, study and much diligence, to labour commendably, and with a good conscience to worke in the Vineyard of Chyrurgery: yet I know there be many young Students in the Arte, will be alwaies ready, and most willing to discharge their dutyes in such matters as they shall take vpon them to deale in, whether it be in this kind of cure, or otherwise. And also will be very carefull, not onely for conscience sake, but euen by a naturall desire, to sæke to increase their skill and necessary knowledge, and therefore it is truely said: the good intent of such honest and well meaning persons, requireth a fauourable acceptation, which is as well to be estæmed, as the performance of them that be best able. And these will bee ready to manifest the same by yælding some fruite of their painfull labour and diligence: And now I wil leaue off discoursing, and begin to speake of my determined purpose, and to make the same more plainely knowne, which I haue hæretofore kept secret vnto my selfe: howbeit, the greatest secret that is, may no longer be called a Secret, when the whole multitude is made acquainted with it.

The

of the *Struma.*   9

The Cure of the foresaid Euill is manyfolde: to wit, inwardly and outwardly, and is performed by two speciall remedies: the one Medicinall, and the other Instrumentall, without the which fewe good workes or Cures in Chyrurgery can be brought to perfection: The reason is, because in this Cure, the vncleanenesse of the body is such, which feedes the matter of the disease. Therefore, first of all the matter must be purged, for as it is said, the roote of al the Cure is y̆ wel purging of the body, whereby Nature is the better enabled to expell and vnburden her selfe of many bad and vnprofitable tumours. And now (by the fauour of the learned) I will therefore begin with remedies Medicinall, according to the maner of Method, published by Calmatheus, one whome amongst many other learned men in Phisicke and Chirurgery, I haue obserued most diligently, as it were a Day-starre or Chrystallin cleare looking glasse, following him with feruent zeale and earnest desire: by reason (as it seemeth vnto me) he was not ignorant in any thing that might make for the truth of his writing, chiefly for the Cure of the foresaid Euill. Yet (I protest) I am no such deuote fauorite of his, or any other mans whatsoeuer, further then iustly they haue deserued: which is the onely cause that hath mooued mee to haue a reuerent estimation of him and all other learned men, whether they doe remaine beyond the Sea, or otherwise abide with vs at home.

Now followeth the maner of Method, by Phi- Struma. sicall remedies for the Cure of Struma, or the Euill which our Kings or Queenes haue and doe still Cure: the experimentall proofe thereof I haue often times seene effected: wherefore I will be short, and presently procede vnto the first intention.

C The

The Artificiall Cure

The first Intention Phisicall by Inward meanes.

He first Intention (after Calmatheus) in the 12. Chap. of his book, for the general cure of Vnnaturall Tumours, is that the curing of this disease called Struma, doth consist in Dyet that dryeth moderately, & heateth and attenuateth the humours: Hunger is profitable, and fulnes is hurtfull: Sleep and Idlenes are euill: exercise before meate very good: the vse of Sulphure or Alume water, is very good and profitable.

The second Intention Phisicall by Inward meanes.

The second Intention is the vse of breaking, attenuating, mundifying & opening Medicaments; as are these Remedies now following. viz.

Recipe. Rad, Ireos. Cort. Sambucj. Boiled in white wine, then adde vnto this decoction, a quantity of Ginger. For this decoction breaketh, attenuateth, openeth & mundifieth dolorous Tumors: so doth it also prouoke vrine, wch in this affect is a speciall matter.

The often vse of the Pilles of Hiera simplex is much commended to cast out Flegme of the stomacke & guts.

But if so be that thou wilt purge the whole body, thou shalt vse the Pilles of Agarico Coccis: if thou list to dissolue & cast out Phlegme, these Pils following must be taken, viz. Pillulæ de Sagap: de Opopan, de Elleboro, de Euphorbio. The Phisitians in times past commended the powder of Turbith, Ginger, and Suger, of each equall parts: The Doses whereof was to two Dragmes.

The

of the *Struma.*

The third Intention Phisicall
by Inward meanes.

The third Intention is the vse of this powder, which doth consume(as they terme it) the Antecedent matter, which it doth aswell by his manifest quality, and (as they say) by a secret property.

This powder doth consume Phlegme, by little & little.

℞. Rad. Aristo. Rotundæ.
    Raphani. } An. ʒ i.
    Spattulæ fœtidæ.
Fol. Pimpinell.
    Pilosell. } An. ʒ ii.
    Rutæ Maioris.
    Scrophulariæ. } An. ʒ. ß.
    Philipend.
    Semen Anisi.   ʒ ii.
    Zingiber.   ʒ i.
    Turbith Optimi } An. ʒ iii
    Sene Orient.
    Saccari Albissimi.   ʒ iii.

Make all these into powder, and let the Patient take euery day in the morning a Spoonefull, with white Wine, or the water of Broome.

  Guido taketh the forenamed powders, and boyleth them in white Wine vntill halfe, & giueth euery third day one quarter thereof.

  Galen approueth & commendeth the vse of Theriaca Vetus, Athanasia et Ambrosia. The vse of Aurea Alexādrina for the cōforting of ỹ stomack, is very good. Also it is said

The Artificiall Cure

that Theriaca Athanasia doe both resolue, breake and digest humours, being compact and gathered together in the profundity of the body.

Purging of childrē after Mercurialis. Mercurialis saith moreouer, that about the purging of children (which is diligently to be obserued) the state of children is weake, that it must bee handled with verie gentle medicines, & rather to be often repeated, & more easier then to minister any stronge Medicines: therfore the belly shall thus be mollifyed.

℞. Mellis Rosatj. ʒ.iii.
  Decoctionis fructuum. ʒ. i. ⎱ Misce.
  Foliorum Senæ. ʒ, ii. ß.   ⎰

But that the humours may be prepared, it must bee done with this Medicine.

℞. Folior. Scrophulariæ
  Plantaginis.
  Betonicæ.   ⎱ Ana. M. ß.
  Menthæ.   ⎰

Make a Decoction according to Arte, and then take of the said Decoction ʒ. j. Syrupj Rosatj recentis, Oxymel. simplisis Ana. ʒ. ß. Mingle these: When the humours bee prepared, they may be purged with this Medicine.

℞. Agaricj Trochiscat. ʒ. j. ⎱
  Squinantj. gra. ij.   ⎰

Steep them in Betony water and straine them. and put thereto.

℞. Mellis Rosatj solutiuj. ʒ. ii.
  Electuarii de Psylio. ʒ. i.
  Decoctionis Cordialis ⎱ ʒ. i.
  Polipodio.   ⎰ ʒ. ii.

Thus much as concerning this briefe note, or compendious Methode of the forensmed Authors, which may very well serue for a very fit President or beginning

of the Struma. 13

ning to the rest that followeth: Now it remaineth that I make heere also report of the singular and rare efficacy of our manuel operation therunto annexed and belonging, with the right vse of the topicall or outward remedies, which is to be externally applyed. The reason is, because it is referred vnto the skilfull Chirurgians manuell or handy working, for the Cure of this great Infirmity, which doth outwardly affect the superficiall parts of the body.

For (as saith Iacobus Ruffus) that to the perfection and accomplishing of the foresaid Cure (called, The Euill by the King, or Queene Cured) he doth reduce it into sixe Intentions Chirurgicall, as followeth. The experimentall verifying of his excellent skill in this disease, as also in many others, is by divers worthy men often times commended: which Malady doth vexe and trouble most pittifully the common sort of people.

The first Intention is, In Attritione, et Compressione.	1
The second Intention is, In Discussione, et Resolutione.	2
The third Intention is, In Suppuratione et Maturatione.	3
The fourth Intention is, In Incisione et Extractione.	4
The fitt Intention is, In Corrosione et Mundificatione.	5
The sixt Intention is, In Obligatione et Evultione.	6

Iacobus Rufus his 6. Intentions chirurgicall, by outward meanes.

ALso (after Fuchsius and other learned men) it is accordingly to be vnderstood as followeth: who also hath written of these Phlegmaticall or Glandulous abcessions called Struma.

If

The Artificiall Cure

If (say they) these abscessions that bee seated in the stronge parts of the body, and because they are not yet olde and inueterate, hauing a thin Cystis that couereth them: these are to be appeased and consumed, and after dryed vp.

The first Intention Chyrurgicall by outward meanes.

Ow I will set downe Examples and Instances for the Cure of the said Malady, the which I haue obserued and gathered (as heereafter ensueth) for the perfection and accomplishing of the before named first Intention, if the strength and ability of the Patient will serue and admit the same. Then one chiefe thing (as you are before tolde) is, that the Patient doe kéep a thin & sparing dyet, which is the efficient cause belonging vnto Phisick. The reason is, as I haue noted, that those which are thus affected, haue alwaies a great inclinatiō to a grosse disordered liberty of fæding: Therefore the Patient must be sustained with such meates, as are agréeable to Nature, and to eschew such meates which make grosse Iuyce: and not (as it is said) to lay gorge vpon gorge. And further yée shall note, though it bee said before, that abstinence is greatly to be commended: yet you must consider it is not meant, that Nature should thereby bee enfæbled, or ouerthrowne, and that especially in weake bodyes, great care must be had: But onely to kéepe all possible abstinence, that is to eate and drinke sparingly and measurably, onely to preserue the strength, and to satisfie Nature: I meane, that it bee such as is agréeable to the strength of the Patient, and
greatnes

of the *Struma*.

greatnes of the Infirmity.

Likewise it is said, the often vse of purging and bléeding on both the Armes, is profitable. Also, it is auaileable to vse Frictions, Rubbings, Borings, and Blisterings is much praised after purgings, for it stoppeth the flowing matter (being applyed vpon the head) by reuulsion or drawing back, & causeth euacuatiõ. Moreouer, it is said, ỹ to discusse these kinds of Tumours which are found in moueable parts, & superficially lodged néer vnto the outward parts, A plate of Leade is most familiar therfore, especially in young persons, by reason of the raritye and softnes of the skinne: It is thought vnfit (by diuers learned men) to blister Childrens heads with Cantharides, it hath béen séene to cause much paine and pissing of bloud: but to doe it by abuisement, either with Mustard or with Nettles, is good. *Mercurialis cõdemneth this course, rather commending Flamula louis, or such like.*

Also, many learned men, of a certaine knowledge and sound vnderstanding, haue in their bookes greatly commended a playster made thus: Recipe. Olde dryed Goates dung, Hony and Vineger, being decocted at an easie fire, to the consistence of a playster. Also, Doues dung mingled with Hony, hath the same effect. So is it by me also wel approoued, this plaister called Oxicroceum, whose composition is not far to be sought for.

℞. Ceræ, Picis, Colophen, Croci.   An. ʒ. iiii.
   Terebinth, Galbanũ, Ammoniaci. ⎫
   Mastici, Olibanum.   ⎬ An. ʒ. j ʒ. iiij.

Dissolue the Gums in Vineger, and powder that which is to be powdred, & so make a plaister according to Arte: Also a plaister of Figs baked and spred, and so applyed vpon Struma is approoued good.

Likewise, Oleum Cucumiris Asininus, dropped into the eare, on that side where the Struma is, is most effectuall to disperse and dissolue.

In like maner, is generally commended Emplastrũ de Ranis

Ranis cum Mercurio, to be appropriate and respectiue in this Cure, to consume superfluous humidity, engendring this disease.

Howbeit, vpon a time a certaine repyning enuious man, being full gorged with a malicious rayling spirit, being proudely giuen (in the gall of much bitternesse, with many scandalous words, and bragging comparisons ill beseeming his person) reported that the aforesaid plaister De Ranis was dangerous vnto the patient; and said, who so did holde the contrary opinion, it was erroneous, foolish and deceiptfull: by reason (quoth hee) of the coldnes of the Quick-siluer: and boldly did seeme to maintaine the same, with a number of very spruse termes, and picked phrases, like as young Children vse to doe, when (in mockery) they counterfeite a strange kinde of language, & forsooth placed them as it were in Geometrical proportions, as though he had bin the onely Son of Archimedes that great Geometritian. In deed it is a most true saying: That fish which is bred in the durt will alwaies taste of the Mud: And I told him that I neuer yet found any more coldnes in this Playster, then there is heate in a paynted fire. But this I doe speake vpon mine owne knowledge, that there is as much difference in Arte and Judgement, betweene this odde fellow (which would seeme to bee a second Æsculapius) and a man replenished with true knowledge indeed, as is betweene a Master Cooke and a Scullian of a Kitchin. Howbeit, hee said also, that his skill was such, that if a man were wounded at Yorke, bring him the weapon that hurt the Patient, and he would cure him (forsooth) by onely dressing of the weapon, and though he neuer see the Patient. As certaine as the Sea burnes. And now heere I will surcease to speake any further of these matters, for I regarded not such sayings, sith it is truely said; Euery man must yeeld an accompt, both of

his

Such is the impudency of bolde blindnes.

of the *Struma*.   17

his case, and of his labour. Themistocles, a Captaine of the Grecians (as Historians make mention) supposed it better to be enuyed of the malicious, then to liue in Idlenes and basenes of minde, without doing some good for the benefit of his Country and Common wealth, wherein he was borne and bred. Now to the second Intention, and so in order with the rest as they doe lye, and offer themselues vnto vs.

Scientia non habet inimicum nisi ignorantem.

The second Intention Chyrurgicall by outward meanes.

THe second Intention Chirurgicall, is the right vse of those remedies which doe mollifye, discusse and consume great abscessions, which are not yet hard and inueterate.

And that the same is true, may easily be gathered as followeth. And for that I wold haue this second Intention made plaine (as much as in me lyeth) and also familiarly knowne vnto the studyous Reader: I doe therfore say, It is meete and conuenient, that those Medicamentes which are to bee vsed, be of the Nature and property to mollifie and discusse, and so to open the powers of the skinne by eusporating, breathing and scattering abroad, and make thinne the grosse matter and Phlegme. Then for the better performance thereof, without further discoursing, I will heere presently set downe (as it were) a Store-house of diuers and sundry approoued Chirurgicall remedyes, necessary for the curing and safe healing of the forenamed Strumacie and Phlegmaticall sicknesse: The which from time to time I haue by experience (the Mistris of all Artes and Sciences) carefully obserued, and faithfully also collected out of the famous writtinges of sundry worthy Authors,

Montanus supposeth these Strumous Tumours somtime to proceede from melancholy

D

thors, as also out of the fruitefull labours, of diuers men famous in experience: whose painfull trauailes and studyes, haue (at this day) most excellently refined this worthy Arte of Chyrurgerie from Barbarisme: otherwise it is greatly to be feared, a number at this day had not béen so skilfull and rich in knowledge, and otherwise, as they are said to be. Therefore we ought not to thinke any study, paines, or trauaile too great, wherein we hope of much benefit to our patients, and also profit and commodity to our selues: And héere I must néeds say, (according to my poore ability) I haue my self béen very industrious for the common benefit, and good of others, truly to set downe diuers approued remedies of mine own collection: wherin (to my knowledge) I haue not in al this whole discourse, published any superfluous and vnapproued remedies, or otherwise kept backe any worthy secret I had: but as did the Euangelicall and heauenly womā mentioned in ye Scriptures, who presented into the Lords Treasury al ye wealth & substance she had. Notwithstanding, I haue read ye men in times past did with great care & diligence consecrate & kéep secret (as a precious treasure vnto thēselues) al such chosen & peculiar remedies, wh they had experienced & approoued for the curing & healing of any dangerous malady: and (as it is said) bound themselues by oath one to another, not to bewray their Secrets by their bookes or writings. Howbeit, I more regarding the publick vtility & good of posterity, did wh great care & diligence consider with my self, what profit can there be to any mā to bury his labors in the lake of obliuion, or otherwise to hide it in the denne of darkenesse. And although I know the matter héer spoken of, may séeme a paradox to some, & so of smal worth: neuerthelesse, although I am none of the greatest Clarks, yet I know it wil be more auailable, then some happily doe make account of. For which cause I haue laboured wh as much perspicuity &
\hfill plainnes

plainnes, as possible I could, to deliuer the truth of my honest & faithful good meaning, so far forth as God hath enabled me in knowledge, skil & memory. Wherefore I meane heere presently to make publicke & open testimony of the same, though now and then I make a little digression, and swarue from my matter, by reason of certaine Crosbyters, who haue heertofore (behinde my backe, and to my face also) not a little abused me: Howbeit, I wil heere conclude this discourse concerning this Second Intention Chirurgicall, & doe confesse and considerately affirme, that there is but few mens labors at the first made so perfect, but that in processe of time & further consideration, they may be bettered, corrected and amended. Yet I cannot but much maruaile, that wise men now a daies are growne to this passe, that they do so seriously follow exorcismes and the Illusions of certaine Charmes of Clowtes and Rags, which is very inhumane and barbarous; neuer practised, neither written of, nor allowed by any learned Phisitiō or Chirurgian that euer I yet heard or read of. Howbeit, the world is (as it were) led in a stringe & carried away to beleeue these vanities, which make a shadow or shew of verity for the safe curing of diuers maladies, & sildome (they say) misse not: But I know the contrary is true, for I haue cured both old & young persons, when these Charmers of clowtes & rags, with their incredible operations haue failed them, & proued flat foolery & absurdities. But to leaue this new Leach craft, with their doting inuentions, I wil here speake of diuers remedies very respectiue & appropriate, for the cure of the before named infirmity, as a president and example for young practizers of Chirurgery to follow. Now vnto the said Second Intention, which is first to set downe those special remedies, whose properties are to open the pores of the skin, & to soften the hard parts, by insencible transspiration.   D 2   A

The Artificiall Cure

A choyse and speciall mollyfying and resoluing plaster, and serueth well for the curing of this græuance: As my selfe haue many times approoued.

Iacobus Ruffus.

℞. Serapini.   ʒ iiii.
   Ammoniaci.   ʒ iii.
   Bdellij.   ʒ i.
   Galbani.   ʒ i.
   Euphorbij.   ʒ ii.

Let these be dissolued in good Malmesey, and then adde thereunto.

Ol. Lilior.   } An. ʒ i.
Ol. Amigdalar. }
Propoleos.   ʒ iiii. ß.
Misce, fiat Implastrum.

Another.

Clowes.

℞. Galbani.   }
   Ammoniaci.   } An. ʒ iii.
   Picis Albæ.   }
   Ceræ Citrinæ. ʒ iiii.
   Ol. pedis Vaccini. q. s.
   Misce.

I doe many times instéd of the Oyle, take the Marow: Then what profit doth ensue, time will approue the same.

Another.

Haly the Abbot.

℞. Farinæ fabar. } An. ʒ. v.
   Farinæ Hord. }
                           Liqueritiæ.

of the *Struma*.

Liqueritiæ,
Rad. Althææ.   } An. ʒ x.
Picis.

Ceræ Albæ.   } An. ʒ x.
Adipis Anserini.

Let there be added the Urine of a Boy, and of olde Oyle q s. And so boyle it to the forme of a Plaister.

Another.

℞. Gum. Ammoniaci.   ℔. ß.   *Banister.*
Rad. Brioniæ in pul.   ʒ j.
Turp. Mineralis.   ʒ i.
Cinnabrij.   ʒ x.
Ceræ.   ʒ ii.

Let the Gumme Armoniacke bee dissolued in Vineger, according to Arte, and after made vp in rowles. Among a number of his memorable deedes, which hee hath left vnto the minde and memory of posterity, this his Plaister deserueth great commendations.

Another.

Mercurialis commendeth a Playster made of Lyme *Mercurialis.* and Salt-Petre, of each like much, being mixed with Barrowes greace. q. s. But such remedyes are too stronge for Children, least it cause Agues, and hurt the soft and tender flesh of their bodies, (chiefly about the Necke) it is to be auoyded. Moreouer, I read, that to make a Playster of Nitrum and Lyme, of each a like quantity, and of Cardamonium & Fenygreeke 4. times so so much, and with Hony make hæreof a Plaister.

Ætius

Ætius saith, when Struma beginneth in children, they must be molifyed and dispersed: And for mollifying in children is approoued this remedy following.

℞. Diachylon.   ℨ iiii.
   Oesypi.   ℨ i.
   Radicum Ireos   ⎱
   Pulueriset.   ⎰ ℨ iiii.

Misce.

Another.

Recipe. The Lées of white or red wine, & of strong Vineger, of each a quart: Mallowe leaues 4. good handful: Boile them till the leaues bee tender, then stampe the leaues, & put them againe into the said licour, with halfe a pound of sweet butter: of barley meale & of beane meale, of each a good handfull: Of Linséede & Fenigrek of each 4. ounces: Of the powder of red Rose leaues one good handfull: Of yolkes of Egges 3. or 4. an of Saffron the waight of 3. d. fiat cat ap las.

I might easily bring in a confused number of other remedies to the same end & purpose, out of diuers learned mens writings, which heer to repeate were needles, and to no great vse, sith I know these may suffice: Wherefore I thinke it good to pretermit the nominating of the rest, &c.

The third Intention Chyrurgicall
by outward meanes.

The third Intention is, to ripen, open and clense such Phlegmaticall Corruptions and Ulcerous Apostumes, which do pertaine to Suppuration: This néedeth no long discourse, sith it plainely appear-

of the *Struma*. 23

eth, that these troublesome, hard kernelly swellings, be found so rebellious, that they doe resist all emollientes and Diaphoreticall remedies before named: by meanes wherof it can not be dissolued & consumed as we happily would, or do desire. For which causes we are further constrained to alter our course, with due consideration, that is to wit: Not to leaue the Patient helples, but to vse stronger Medicamentes, I meane Suppuratiues, as is before said, such as whose property is to bring superfluous humours to maturity and ripenes, by these and such like Emplasticke remedies, which (as it is said) doe by the closing of the pooers of the skin, augment the naturall heate, whereby the matter so enclosed causeth the generatiō of matter or Pus. But I must confesse, I haue not often times séene these hard Phlegmaticall abcessions easily brought to suppuration. The matter being once colde, dull, Clammy, hard and knotty, and déeply seated, and of a long continuance in a body, whose skin is grosse and thicke, & the matter hardly compact: These kindes (I haue found) do sildome come to maturity and ripenes, vnlesse (as Cornelius Celsus saith) the said Tumours bée mixed and made of matter and bloud. And Trincauel reporteth, that some of these Tumours that haue heate in them, doe ripen and come to matter & suppuration: But there be others that be more hard, and doe resist suppuration, and then they come néerer vnto the nature of a Scirrhus. Now it followeth that I set downe those approoued remedies, being in vulgar vse, seruing for suppuration, which are long agoe ratifyed and well allowed of, by a vniforme consent, both of olde & late wryters, which were men of an industrious capacity, & of a most rare & exquisite knowledge in the Arte. And first I wil begin with Iohannes de Vigo, one of the chief Fathers, & true Patrones of al good learning & knowledge in the Arte of Chirurgery:

Nota

As

The Artificiall Cure

Nota.

As it (in some sort) may appeare by Master Bartholmew Traheron, which first Translated Vigo in the English tongue. In his Epistle Dedicatory (whose iudgement therein I doe acknowledge) hee sayth: that although Vigo were not brought vp in the knowledge of the Tongues, yet through his singular wit, long experience, and diligent study, hee hath inuented and set foorth, more notable things in the Arte of Chirurgerie, then any other héeretofore: and I thinke sayth he, nothing can better testifye the cunning of this man, then that he continued so long in Rome, in such a company of pocky Curtezans: neither Priests, Bishops, nor Cardinals excepted, as it appeareth in his Booke: for where such cariones béen, the best Egles will resort, &c.

A Maturatiue Playster.

℞.   Radices Althææ.   } Ana. ℔.ß.
     Capit. Liliorum.

Let these boyle in a sufficient quantity of Water, and after being stamped, put vnto them of Garlicke and white Onions roasted, vnder the coales of each. ʒ iij.

Vigo.

Ol. Liliorum.   } An. ʒ ii.
Butyri.

Pinguedinis porcini.   } An. ʒ. ii. ß.
Anserinæ.

Farinæ Tritici.   } An. q. s.
Fenigreci.

Make a Playster at the fire, adding in the ende, the yolkes of two Egges: There bee some (I know) doe little

of the *Struma*.

little prize or value this Playster, but I doe acknowledge it to be an infallible remedy.

Another.

℞. Radices Bryoniæ.	℔. ß.	D. F.
Ceparum.	No. ii.	
Rad. Althææ recentiũ.	ʒ. iiii.	
Fol. Maluarum siccarum.	p. i.	
Hidropiperis.	M. i.	
Ficuum.	} An. ʒ j.	
Passularum Enucleatarum.		

Boyle them well, then adde vnto them.

Fermenti.	} An. ʒ ii.
Axungiæ suillæ Insulsæ.	
Euphorbij. pul.	ʒ i.

Misce et fiat Emplastrum secundum artem.

This playster worketh miraculous effectes in this Cure.

Another Playster.

℞. Mirrhæ.	ʒ x.	Paulus Aegineta.
Ammoniaci Thymiamatis.	ʒ vii.	
Visci Quercini.	ʒ viii.	
Galbani.	ʒ iiii.	
Propolis.	ʒ i.	

Misce et fiat Emplastrum secundum Artem.

A Maturatiue Cataplasme.

Recipe. Rye-bread lib. i. White Onions & of Lilly rootes

ly Rootes, roasted vnder the Ashes, of each 4. Ounces. A Bryony Roote, and Figges boyled in Malmesey, of each 6. Ounc. Fenygreke & Lynseede, of each 3. Dun. Barlye meale and Beane meale, of each 4. Dun. Oyle of Roses, Camomill and Wormewood, of each 3. Dun. Hony 4. Dun. The yolkes of 4. Egges hard roasted. Saffron the waight of 4. d. Boyle all these together to a laudable consistence, and apply it thicke vnto the grieued partes, morning and euening warme.

This medicine Mercurialis alloweth likewise. cap. de Struma.

Also I read in Iohannes Libaulty, his Booke Instituted Le Meson Rustick, and also in other Learned Writers, that the dung of a Cow heated vnder the Ashes, betwixt Uine or Colwort leaues, & mingled with vineger, hath the property to bring Scrophulous swellings to ripenes, &c. Nothwithstanding, if all these chaunce to faile, then haue recourse to that which followeth in the Fourth Intention, which is perfomed by Section or Incision, when wee finde the matter before rehearsed, vnfit to yeeld eyther to Resolution or Suppuration, &c,

The fourth Intention Chyrurgicall
by outward meanes.

THe fourth Intention of these Strumous Tumors, which are not cured by former remedies (& yet are gentle, obedient and tractable) is to cut them off, and then to pull them out.

In the vse of these outward Incisions, this scope ought chiefly to be regarded, that is: to be very circumspect in your handy operations, attempted & done cocerning the cure of this great Malady: That is, the apertion or opening by launcing or Incision of those glandulous Tumors. For as it is said, bloud is the treasure of life, and habitation of the soule: Moreouer, it is surely very hard and difficult, especially when there is in the affected place, eyther Nerue, great Uaine, or Artery, &c.

There

of the *Struma*.

Therefore such persons as are to endure this painfull action, ought to haue much patience, and to be of a good courage: Then it may bee the better attempted and done by a cunning and skilfull Chyrurgian: which there is no doubt, but he will be so prouident, that nothing shall offend. How be it, it is not necessary or sufferable ouer curiously to search and attempt the cutting them out by Incision: For that many of them are subiect to violent and inordinate bloudy Fluxes, and other euill accidents, which doubtlesse will much amaze you and hinder your handy operation: I meane, when these Tumors bee déeply planted, and secretly lodged amongst the great vaines and Arteries called Carotides, or otherwise néere the Nerui recurrentes, which is often times the cause that some bee come spéechlesse thereby. And it cannot be iustly denyed, but that these Incisions haue often times béen attempted with a launce by our Ancestors & Fore-fathers. But amongst a number of those worthy men, Wickar being a man of good knowledge & skill in the Cure of the foresaid Euill, his counsaile is, that before we doe attempt the said action by Incision, the Patient be first layde vpon his Bed, and so both his féet must be strongly tyed vnto the bed poasts, his head & both his hands must also be fast held by men of strength, and skilfull in holding: In such sort as we doe in cutting those which haue the crooked or wrye neckes. And he that is chosen to be the Operator of the said action, must prudently and wisely (saith Vigo, and other learned men) cósider the greatnes & smalnes of the said Tumor, which must be incised & cut fró one length of the Tumor to an other. Then by litle & litle, seperate, diuide & vndermine the whole Cistis round about, to the very bottome & roots therof, not rashly, nor by violence, but orderly by degrées, seperate w your fingers, & other seruiceable instrumēts, as you vse to diuide ỹ forenamed

Wennes

Wennes called Steatoma, Atheroma and Meliceris: And confessed it is for a certaine, that if any portion or part of the said Cistis or bagge, chaunce to remaine behinde, and not cleare taken away by the rootes, it will (doubtlesse) breed and increase againe: But to preuent such greeuances, me thinkes I cannot speake too sufficietly therof: wherfore, if any part remain behinde, then lay vpon it the powder of Mercury precipitate, or (if that bee too weake) adde to it of Alumen Combust, or Vitriolum Album combust, of each equall portions: notwithstanding I beleeue, & confidently hold, that the worke of your hands is the best instruments you haue to trust to, and to relieue you in this distresse.

Mercurialis.   Moreouer, Mercurialis he further sayth these words, for the curing and effecting of this matter: First (saith he) chuse some light place, & let the Patient lye on his bed, for in sitting he wil soone sound: therfore binde his legges together, and after binde them to the Bedside, and let one holde his head fast, and then the Chirurgean taking the swelling in his left hand, let him make an Incision, eyther right or straight, or somewhat crooked, on the necke vnder the Jaw-bones, vntill he come to the matter inclosed in the Bladder, which is sometimes one and single, as in the lesser swellinges, and sometimes double, like the Myrtle leafe in the greater swellinges: So that conueniently (eyther by the fingers or other Instrumentes) the Bladder may bee by little and little separated, and drawne from the next partes, together with the matter inclosed in it. But take good heede that the Bladder be not cut, because it is hardly drawne away, and much hindreth the Cure, and the euill will come againe: But if any such thing chaunce, it were good to consume it with eating Medicines. Great care must also be had, that neyther the Arteries, vaines, nor notable Nerues be hurt, but by little

and

and little gently put it aside. Yet if in the cutting some vessell be diuided, and the issue of bloud trouble and hinder the worke: then apply some meete thing to stay the bloud, and so come againe to your worke: For if the lippes of the Incision be inflamed, and the swelling or Struma bee not safely dissolued away: then lay on a Stupa beaten with the White of an Egge, and such things as be good for stopping of bloud. After, apply Medicines that wil a little concoct, and then vse abstersiues, and next such as causeth fleshe to growe and heale vp the scarre.

The fifth Intention Chyrurgicall by outward meanes.

The fifth Intention is, those which are vnmoueable, and deepely rooted within, Corrode them about and clense them throughly. I graunt it tollerable and very conuenient, to vse in this Cure the due applycation of Potential Cauteries, such as whose propertye and seruice is to corrode the flesh & the skin, and may with very good circumspection very safely be attempted, being administred vpon a body that is of a reasonable constitution, & in such sort that his strength is able to holde and endure the same. And hære I will make further demonstration thereof, that is to say: that your Cautery be not applyed vpon any Sinnewy part, neither vpon the great Vaines nor Arteries, for that these bee accompted indæde principall and chiefe vessels: Also you must consider the quallity and quantity of the Causticke you doe administer, for that some are more violent and stronger then other, and some wil run and spread more then another.

Iaques Guillemeau Chyrurgian vnto the now French King

King which now is: saith, truely it is not necessary, nor allowable to apply the Caustick vpon the endes or beginnings of Muscles, for if your Patient that is to bee Cauterized, haue an vnsound and sickly body, you must first of all bee sure before you administer the sayd Cautery, to Phlebotomize & purge him: The reason is, least in the Cauterized parts, there chaunce to come concursion, or gathering together of humours. Also, it is further sayd, that a small part of your potentiall Cauteryes, doth and will worke as forcibly on a soft and tender bodye, as a great quantity thereof will doe vpon a stronge and grosse obdurate person. Ouer and besides, the greater abcessions are to bee Cauterized one way, and the lesser an other way, and that with good consideration. And heere to put you in memory, that you must bee very carefull and circumspect in defending the partes round about the sayd Tumors, for feare (as I haue said) that your Cautery doe run and spread too farre abroad: for the which cause you shall strengthen, fortifye & defend the foresaid affected parts, that is to say: by inuironing and compassing it round about with some repercussiue Medicamentes, lest the grieued part (which by long infirmity is become thereby sore weakned & enfeebled) and may so bring with it great swelling & other euill accidents: And therfore it is not without good cause, that the parts grëeued be rightly ordred & defended, whereby you shall be sure the better to effect your intended purpose without the said perill or daunger but with the highest commendation in preuenting the euill that otherwise might ensue: which reasons alwaies enduced mee to laye round about the Cauterized parts, some speciall defensiue, as is this, or the like hëereafter following.

A good defensatiue. Reci. Emplastrum Diachalcithios dissolued in Ol. papaueris et Ol. ros. wherunto is added Ouorum albumin,

of the *Struma*.

min.et Aceti.rof. An.q.s.
  Et fiat Emplaſtrum.

This done, then preſently goe about with your Cauſticke, to roote out all the whole Schrophulous and hard kernelly ſubſtances, either with the common Ruptory or Cauſticke, which in this caſe beſt contenteth my minde: the making hæreof I doe not hære ſet downe, becauſe it is ſo commonly knowne.

Howbeit, there is an other Cauſticke, which (as it is reported vnto me by a ſkilful Chirurgian) doth worke without any paine, or very litle at al. The reputed Author therof is ſaid to bee a famous practizer in Chirurgery, dwelling at Mountpelier in France. I muſt néedes thinke reuerently of the Author of this Cauſtick, hoping his minde was not ſuch to delight himſelfe with publiſhing of vntruth: But if it doe indéede worke without paine, the miſtery thereof is farre aboue my reach.

Rec. Lixiuij Saponarij.   lib ij.
     Vitriolj Romanj.   ℥ iij.
     Mercurij ſublimatj.   ℥ j.

Made into very fine powder: in the end of the boyling put in of Opium 2.drams. Miſce et fiat Trochiſci.

A good potentiall Cautery:

You ſhall further note, that if at any time your Cauſticke doe happen not to worke ſo well and ſufficiently to your minde, as happily you would wiſh it ſhould do, then apply the ſame Cautery againe: but you muſt firſt make Inciſion alongſt wiſe, vpon the middle of the foreſaid Eſcharre: Then put in ſome ſmall quantity (that is, ſo much as you ſuppoſe will penetrate into the profundity & very rootes therof) for it doth behoue a prouident & wiſe Artiſt to preuent & ſée all eminent danger in ẏ doing thereof, & thē by Gods help, ye may ſafely in a ſhort time roote out theſe hard Strophulous Tumors. For (as I haue ſaid) vnleſſe the roote be cleane takē out,

this

this Malady will growe and increase againe. But if there chaunce to approach any painefull accidentes (as I haue knowne and seene to follow in sundry persons) then with speed remooue and take away the same: which done, yee shall procure the fall of the Eschar, with Vnguentū Populeum: or els with Vnguentum Rosarum, or sweete Butter. And to apply vpon it Emplastrum Diacalcitheos, or Emplastrum Deminio. So after all the Escharres be remooued, then if there be required mundifying and clensing, these following are vulgarly vsed, as Vnguentum Apostolorū, called of some also Vnguentum Christianorū: which Vnguent in this effect cannot be bettered: and Vnguentum Egiptiacum, and sometimes to mixe two parts of Vnguentum Apostolorum, and one part of Vnguentum Egiptiacum. Also, Vnguentum Apij, is auaileable in this Cure, viz.

Vnguentū ex Apio.

Recipe, Succi Apij et Plantaginis.   An. ℥ ij.
   Farinæ hordej et Orobj. An ℥ j. ß.
   Terebinthinæ,   ℥ j.
   Mellis,   ℥ iij.
   Mirrhæ   ℨ iij.
  Misce et fiat Vnguentum.

If you adde to this Vnguent the yolkes of Egges and Mercury Præcipit. it doth worke much better. Also the powder of Mercury præcipit. is good of it selfe, and if you will haue it worke more forcibly, adde vnto it of Allum combust according to discretion. With these foresaid remedyes you may continue vntill there appeare pure and quicke flesh: then it followeth to vse Incarnatiues, & Agglutinatiues, with other medicamēts, fit for consolidation.

Thus hauing sufficiently intreated of the fifth Intention: now it remaineth for a full conclusion, to present

sent in order last of all, the sixt Intention, as followeth.

The sixth Intention Chyrurgicall
by outward meanes.

The sirt Intention Chirurgicall is, that in those Strumas that are fastened but to a thinne and slender roote, you shall binde them about and plucke them out. This last action (as it appeareth) is verie easily performed by a skilfull Operator or cunning Chirurgian: neyther doth it require any great curiosity, but a decent and artificiall strong binding, meete for the plucking of them out (as it is said) by the rootes. In which action you neede not feare any great perrill of Fluxe of bloud, but that it may easily bee restrained with my restringent powder, published in my last booke of Obseruations, which hath (of a number of good Artistes) a friendlye acceptation: If it chaunce through the ill disposition of the body, any dolorous accidentes doe happen to follow, then mitigate the same (sayth Wicker) with stupes wet in the white of an Egge, and oyle of Roses: and afterwards if there growes filthynes, let it be clensed with those remedyes before rehearsed: then no fault being committed through negligence or want of skill, you shall no doubt with good successe, finish this last Intention. But amongst a number of excellent remedyes for the curing of this euill (after the partes bee throughly clensed from all annoyances) this Playster following hath all the properties, that is prescribed in these kindes of remedyes before named: Which noble Playster I obtained of one Isack a stran- M. Isackes ger borne, a famous Incisioner and Licentiate Chi- Playster. rurgian of London, who for his excellent knowledge in

F his

his Arte, was called beyond the Seas, The golden Master or Doctor.

R. Bdellii, et Ammoniaci. An. ʒ i.ß.
Lapidis Sanguinalis, lapidis Magnetis. An. ʒ i.ß
Aristolochiæ rotundæ, aloes Hepaticæ. An. ʒ iii.
Olibanj et Masticis. An. ʒ i.
Lithargirij argēt. et lapidis calaminaris. An. ʒ iii
Corallj Rubj et albi. An. ʒ ii.
Lumbricorum in pul. ʒ j.
Succj scrophulariæ. ʒ vj.
Colophoniæ. ℔ ß.
Terebynthiæ Venetæ. ʒ iiij.
Ceræ Albæ. ʒ xii.
Olej Hispanicj.
Olej Hipericj cum gummis. } An. ʒ iii
Olej Laurini
Camphor. ʒ ß.
  Misce et fiat Implastrum,

With this Playster onely I cured a Bricklayers Daughter neere London, of diuers bad Scrophulous Ulcers in her necke and throate. Howbeit, there be some (who are as it were so nose-wise) that forsooth they can not abide to read any medicine, that is of a long composition, be it neuer so precious. Contrariwise, there be others againe, that will not endure to read a short composition, bee it neuer so well approoued: for they plainely say, there can bee no great matter of worth in them: And thus they are as variable in their opinions (for want of true Arte and iudgement) as the Camelions be in their colours. Quot capita tot sensus: so many heades so many opinions. Now heere I will forbeare

of the Struma.

beare any further to discourse of this Sixt Intention Chirurgicall, but I will set downe certaine Obseruations for the Cure of this grieuous Malady by me perfected, as followeth: least otherwise happily it may bee said, He that telleth a long processe or boasting tedious tale without some proofe, must needs require credit, either for his long boasting tedious tale, or else for some speciall Authority that is in his person. But as for boasting amongst wise men, it can winne litle credit.

An obseruation.

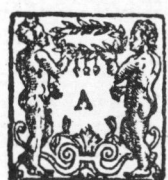

A Few monthes past there was sent vnto me by a Gentleman of Essex, a certaine husband man, being about the Age of thirty yeeres, who was molested (for the space of sixe monthes) with certaine outward swellings, or vnnaturall Strumous Abscessions: some of them were great with notable hardnesses, some meane, and some smaller, being for the most part packed and heaped together, but yet mooued too and fro, hyther and thyther: For the which he was first purged (with great moderation and aduisement) with the pilles of Euphorbium and Trochisce ex Viperis: or the Pilles of Vipers, and he did take many times Theriaca Andromachj, & kept a very slender dyet withall: after hee was well purged from grosse and rawe humours, then I applyed vpon his necke and both his shoulders 3 great cupping glasses, and so did draw bloud and humours in good quantity. After the application of this kinde of Boxing or Ventoses, then presently I applyed vpon his swelling this Vnguent, and these Plaisters following.

Recipe.

The Artificiall Cure

The vnguēt singular good to cōsume all scrophulous Abscessions.

Recip. Colewort leaues, gréene Léekes and blades of water Betonye, Motherwort, the lesse Plantine, Daysie leaues and Flowers, Mallows, Nicotian, and Pelitory of the wall, of each a handfull: Beate and shred these hearbes very fine: then adde to these foresaid hearbes of Wine Wineger lib. ii. of Hogs grease and swéet Butter, of each lib. ii. of oyle of Almonds lib. j. a yong Fox, of earth wormes, & shel snailes, of each lib. i. Let all these lye infused & buryed in horse dung the space of a month, then boyle all together till the watrynes be consumed: then strayne it strongly, & hærewith morning and euening anoynt his necke very warme, for halfe an houre together: Then applyed ℞ Emplastrum de ranis cum Mercurio: and at other times, Emplastrum Dyachilon maius, et de Muscilaginibus, of each equal portions: and by this way and order of curing, he was by me cured and safely healed within the space of 40. dayes.

Another obseruation.

Another obseruation of a Master of a Ship.

Vpon a time there was brought vnto me a certaine Master of a Ship, by a Seruant of mine, called Robert Coulter, a man who (for his knowledge and skill in the Arte of Chirurgery) was greatly estéemed of diuers Nobles, and worthy Persons. This Master of the Ship was mightily infected with many Vlcerous Strumaes in his necke, throate and brest, with much out-growing flesh, loathsome and vnpleasant to beholde: his hard swelling excéeded in number, magnitude and greatnesse: he had a crasie and vnsound body: his minde much troubled with pensiuenesse and melancholy fansies. Cherfore being loath to admit any thing néedfull, or commit any thing

of the *Struma*.

thing hurtfull, I did take the aduise and counsaile of a graue and learned Phisitian: who prepared and purged his body from much crude and rawe indigested excrementall humours, with the Pilles of Sagapenum de Agarico Coctiæ. An ʒ.ß. Misce. In like manner he did set him downe a good regiment of dyet, which was thinne and sparing and light of digestion. He also forbad him eating and drinking at vnaccustomed houres: also he did refraine those meates that were grosse and tough: as Beefe, Milke, fryed Egges, hard cheese, all pulse and nuttes, and other meates which cause thicke Juyce: Also he did appoint him after his first purgings euery morning and euening for a space, to receiue this drinke following, which procured him to auoyde much Phlegmaticke rawe humours, especially by Urine.

℞.	Apij Rusticj et Eupatorij,	An. M. i.	A drinke to procure Vrine.
	Soldanellæ.	M. ii.	
	Petroselini Macedonici.	} An. M. j. ß.	
	Herbæ Trinitatis.		
	Mellis com. lib. ß. Gingiberis.	ʒ ß.	
	Vini Albi et Aquæ com.	An. lib. vi.	
And of fine	Mythridat.	ʒ. iii.	

¶ But be sure yee gather the hearbes when the Sunne is on them, and boyle them to the consumption of the third part, in an earthen pot nealled and close couered, so that no ayre goe foorth: when it is colde, straine it and keepe it in cleane vessels.

And for that this my Patient was subiect to much Restriction of his belly: hee did also admit him to forbeare the foresaid drinke, and to drink of this Laxatiue decoction a quarter of a pinte at a time, which he receiued first in the morning, & at 3. or 4. of the clocke in the

F 3 after-

afternoone, and laſt in the euening.

	℞		
The purging decoction.		Sarſæparillæ.	℥ iiij.
		Rad. ſaſſafras.	℥ ij.
		Ligni ſancti.	℥ iii.
		Epithymi.	} An. ℥ i.
		Hermodactil et	
M. L.		Stechados,	
		Seminis Aniſi.	℥ i.
		Liquerisiæ.	℥ ß.
		Senæ Orientall.	℥ ii.
		Saccari albi.	lib. ß.
		Mithridati.	℥ i.
		Vini albi.	} An. lib. viii.
		Aquæ com.	

Boyle them vnto the third part, and laſt put in your Senæ and Mithridate, and let it not boyle much aboue halfe a dozen walmes. Et fiat.

Local remedyes. Now for that his Vlcers were many, and ſubiect to a hotte diſtemper, for that cauſe hee might the better admitte bloud letting, being alſo a man of a growne age, therefore I tooke the more quantity thereof. Then next I proceeded with the Cure of the beforenamed malignant Vlcers, and did firſt bathe or waſhe them for a good ſpace with Hydromel (that is, Well-water and Hony boyled together) by reaſon of the hotte diſtemperature, and did ſubdue the whole Scrophula, following Vigoes direction: after Inciſion I did put againe of the Cauſticke into the middle of the Carnoſity, which deceiued me not, and ſo after cauſed him to auoyde much noyſome matter and filthyneſſe:

of the Struma. 39

filthines: Then after I did mundifye them with Vnguentum Apostolorum Mesuei, and of Vnguentum Ægiptiacum An. Oun. 2. Oleum Ouorum, Mel Rosarum An. Oun. 2. Lapis Calaminaris preparat made into most subtill powder. Misce et fiat Vnguentum.

I found this aforesaid Vnguent very commodious and profitable in this Cure, and did continue with it till I perceiued pure and quicke flesh: then I did also constitute and ordaine these two remedyes which in their operation for the cure of the said Struma, is approued profitable.

    Recipe. Saccari Plumbj.   ℥. ß.
           Ol. Ouorum lutorum.   ℥ ij.
           Misce.

This place will not admit me heere orderly, to set downe at large, those great cures which I haue seene healed by other Chirurgians, of whome I obtained the knowledge of the foresaid remedyes: And I haue also with the same, cured and healed many of the like cures, but especially in the curing of fraudulēt Vlcers in Ano, the said remedy being Artificially made and prepared according to the Chymistes Arte, the subiect is onely Plumbj rub. et Acetj fort. Also I haue thought it good to set downe the manner of making the foresaid Ol. Ouor. that is: take 20. or 30. Egges, more or lesse, & let them be sodden very hard: which done, lay aside the whites, and reserue onely the yolks, so let them be well laboured and beaten in a cleane morter: then put them into a Frying pan, & cause thē be well fryed, continually stirring them, till it come to an Oylye substance, and after presse it foorth according to Arte.

                                              Recipe.

Recipe. White Varnish.   ℥ ij.
         Lytarge of golde.   ℥ j.

Put the Varnish in a little broad earthen Pan, being made flat and well nealed, the bignes of a great Sawcer, and strewe in the Litarge by little and little, and stir it together euery two houres, and it will in the end come to a certaine hardnesse, in such sort that you may beate it to powder, and strew of this powder vpon your Pledgets, for the cure of ye outward Abscession, which likewise troubled him greatly, being so hard, nody and knotty, so that I feared they would haue degenerate into a Scirrhus, but I did mollify and dissolue them with these remedyes following.

A speciall molifying & dissoluing Cataplasma

G. Kebble.

Recipe. Turnips and Lilly rootes An. lib ß. boyled in stronge Ale or Malmesey, q. s. which being boyled very tender, then straine gently foorth the lyquors, and beate the roote very well in a stone morter, and adde therunto Beane meale and Barly meale, and Ote-meale, of each a handfull: then take the liquors that the fore named rootes were boyled in, and adde thereunto Marsh Mallow rootes two handfuls, of Fenygreke and Lineseede, each of them a handfull. Let these stand infused 12. houres, then boyle it to a thicknesse, and so straine it strongly. Then take of this Mussilage lib. ß. and adde to it also Oyle of Lineseede and sweet Butter An. q. s. and of Saffron the waight of 4. d. Then boyle all together to a consistence. Et fiat Cataplasma.

Also, I often vsed Emplastrum de Ranis cum Mercurio et Emplastrum Dyachilon maius, Emplastrum de Muscilaginibus, as is before named: And thus I cured this Sea-faring man, and so continued (to my knowledge) 11. yeares: in the end hee dyed in the last voyage with Sir Frances Drake.

An

An Obſeruation of a Maide, whoſe friends ſuppoſed ſhe had the Euill before rehearſed, when I was but a young Profeſſor in this faculty and Arte of Chyrurgerie.

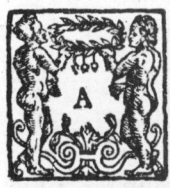

About thirty yéeres paſt (as it were in the minority of this my practice) I did obſerue there was brought vnto me (by a Preacher, then being Vicar of Yalding, a towne in Kent) a Maiden about the age of 22. yeares, hauing a ſtronge and able body, and of a reaſonable good conſtitution, who was ſuppoſed to haue that Euill, called Struma. Yée ſhall vnderſtand, this Vicar was a man that did practiſe both Phiſicke and Chirurgery: this Mayden was a long time troubled with an Vlcer in one of her legges, and a great ſwelling in one ſide of her necke: which Maladyes, the foreſaid Vickar did take vpon him to cure and heale: how be it, in continuance of time he grew weary of his worke, and tolde a neighbour of his, called Maſter Eden (a Gentleman dwelling alſo in Yalding) that the Maide his Patient (as hee ſuppoſed) had the Quéenes Euill (which Gentlemans Daughter not long before I had cured of the ſame:) The ſayd Gentleman perſwaded the Vicar not to ſpend time to long, but to cauſe her to bee ſent vp to London to mee, whoſe counſaile preſently he followed, & the Vicar and the Maide and her father conſulted together, and came to mée to London, and ſhewed me her griefe, and the continuance of the ſame. So after diligent view taken by me, I found it was not the Euil (as ye ſuppoſed) but a ſort

An obſeruation of a Maide dwelling at Yalding in Kent

By the aduice of one M. Archēboule and Beeden Chirurgians of London.

G

a sort of crude and rawe humours, flocking together in her neck, with a putrifyed corrupt Vlcer vpon her right leg, & so I told him he was deceiued in her griefe. Then they went their way and asked further counsell, which all were of my opinion. Then they came vnto me the next day, and I did vndertake the cure with the counsaile of one Doctor Spering a graue and learned Phisition, who prescribed her an order of dyet, with conuenient purging. It is to be noted, hee gaue vnto her in three seuerall boxes, three sundry purgations to be taken at three seuerall times, set downe in writing very plainely, as might be deuised. In like maner I deliuered vnto them all such locall remedies as was fit for both her griefes: amongst the rest I noted in writing, that the first thing shee should vse vnto the Vlcer on her legge, was Vnguentum Ægiptiacum, which I made very strong, and of a high and thicke body, for that I would haue her spred it vpō pledgets somwhat thick, and after to proceede with other meete remedies.

But note what ill hap followed by the Maydes carelesnes, and too much negligence: In the morning after shee came home to Yalding by 7. of the clocke, and tooke one of the 3. Purgations which the Doctor gaue vnto her to take, shee set it vpon a stoole by the fire, where shee meant first to dresse her legge: in conclusion (by great ouersight) she laide the Purgation to her legge, and did eate vp the whole boxe of Aegiptiacum, which was nere 2. oun. and (as she said afterwards) it was very vntoothsome and loathsome in tasting. All this while for two hours space she felt litle working of it, but did begin in the end greatly to burne, & did complaine in her stomacke, throate & mouth, and casted extreamely, & also shortly after purged downe very greatly, & thus continued for the space of one day, & one night before she sought for helpe. In the end, the Vicar was

not

of the *Struma*. 43

not to be found, but ſtayed at London, then they ſent vnto Maideſtone to an Italian Phiſitian called Santa-Ci‑ lia, and he being giuen to vnderſtand by them, that by meanes of a purgation, ſhee was in a great burning heate in her body, & purged & vomitted too aboundant‑ ly, and ſo wanted ſleepe greatly, for the which hee gaue them a preſcript vnto the Apothecary: but firſt that they themſelues ſhould apply her with butter-milke, and new milke, and ſome good fat Mutton brothes: and to helpe to ſtay her purging, he counſailed them to giue her to drinke oftentimes, Red-wine and Conſerue of Sloes together, and to procure her to ſleepe with this potion following.

Santa-Cilia.

℞. Diaſcordij.   ℨ i. ß.
    Diacodij.   ℥ j.
    Aquæ Cardui Benedicti.   fiat potio.

A potion to procure ſleep

But this did ſmall pleaſure. The next night hee ſent her this enſuing.

℞. Diaſcordij.   ℈. iiii.
    Philonij Romanj.   ℈. i.
    Aquæ Cardui Benedicti.   ℥. iii.
    Sir. de Succo Lymonum.   ℥. i.
        Miſce.

Another.

With this ſhe had ſome comfort, but not to that pur‑ poſe they looked for: ſo after the third night, in the next morning they ſent with all ſpeede to my houſe in Lon‑ don with a letter, of the great daunger ſhe was in, & the Phiſitians billes with all what ſhe had done: and pre‑ ſently I ſent it to D. Spering, who was greatly grieued to heare of it, & ſaid he was ſure there was ſome extra‑ ordinary matter in it, for the purgations he ſent would neuer bring her into ſuch danger. Then after he had well conſidered of the matter, & preſent daunger that might

G 2   enſue,

ensue, hee prescribed foorthwith that his Apothecary should make first, for to coole and quench her great and extreame thirst, and to helpe her to her tasting againe, this Iulip which was thus made.

Rec. Barly Water lib. iiii. Conserue of red Roses and of Barberyes, of each 2. Oun: Whereunto was added 20. droppes of Oyle of Vitrioll. Misce.

And then she did drinke for a space, which wrought to good effect in cooling of her, & so brought her to a good taste againe. For the staying of the Fluxe of her Belly and Vomiting, she tooke of this Electuary at diuers times a day, the quantity of 3. Oun. at a time. The making héereof is as followeth.

An Electuary to stay great Fluxes in the Belly.

Recipe. Bol. Armoniacj Orient.   ℥ j.
   Cynamomj.   ℥ j.
   Cloues and Nutmegs roasted.   An. ℥. ß.
   Macis.   ℥ j.
   Sanguinis Hominis, dryed in the Sun, and made into fine powder.   ℥ ij.
   Corticis Balastej.   ℥ j.

Of white Paper shred into a number of small péeces: of Sorrell séedes, and of Plantine séedes, dryed and made into fine powder, of each.   ℥ j.

Boyle these in 12. Oun. of Sirupe of Vineger, till it come vnto the thicknes of an Electuary, &c.

He gaue also vnto her the first night, a Pill of Ladanum, onely to procure sléepe and quiet rest, and caused her to be couered with many cloathes, and so procured sweate: Thus within an houre and a quarter shee fell a sléepe, and rested quietly vntill nine of the clocke the next morning, and neuer casted nor went to the stoole: and (being awaked) confessed shee was greatly refreshed, and felt no paines at all till towards night, and then shee casted a litle, and went now and then to the stoole:

for

for which cause she tooke her fore said Electuary. She earnestly required to haue an other Pill, but the Doctor gaue his direction to the contrary, and would first sée how Nature did dispose her selfe: so the night following she rested but litle, how be it a great deale better then before. Then the third night hee gaue her the second Pill, and after that she neuer vomitted or purged disorderly againe: the excellency of these remedyes is aboue beliefe and vncredible, that I haue done and séen done by these last worthy remedyes, both by Sea and by land The seauenth day after she had receiued her infortunate Purgation of Ægiptiacū, then spéeches was made by me to sée the Vlcer of her legge, but they regarded it not; in the ende she opened it, and found it almost cleane cured, then shee commended mee, and so did her friends for this my excellent remedy: but shee said would neuer take the like Purgation againe, for a thousand pound: thus she was cured by Fortune and not by Arte. Then I required of her, where the Boxes were, that the Purgations and the Vnguentum Aegiptiacum were in? she said she threwe them both into the fire: For (said shee) the Purgation had a filthy taste, and was so clammy, and so sticked to her mouth and téeth, that I had neuer so much a doe (said she) to get it downe my throate. Then I perceiued shee had taken the wrong thing, & it was the more apparant by reason of the blacknes of her téeth, & the staines of her cloathes wherwith she had often wiped her mouth: and also by staining of the Basons and the dishes, wherin she had so often times vomitted. After this I stayed with her ten daies, til her legge and mouth was perfectly cured, and then wee were royally payde, and thus went to London to the Doctor, and tolde him what had hapned, that she had eaten the boxe of Aegiptiacum, and layde the Purgation to her legge, whereat he was greatly grieued:

ued: and much controuersie in spéeches was after betwéene the Doctor and the Maides father, but in the ende they were made friends.

Now I will set downe the composition of the said Pill of Ladanum, which I obtained of a very déere friend, being a pretious Iewell, as it is vsed: otherwise, (as I haue said in other of my writings) the best Medicine that is, is no Medicine vnlesse it be in the hands of a skilfull man.

The true maner and making
of Ladanum.

Take of Opium, first sliced thinne and then dryed in an Earthen platter, one Oun. & a halfe. of the gum of the roote of Henbane 3. Oun. Make the Gum thus. Gather the rootes of white Henbane in March (the Moone being full) and drie them in the shadow: after slice them and boyle them in good white Wine: (the rootes being boyled vntil they be very soft) poure off the wine, being full of the tincture thereof, and presse strongly the rootes, the licour (being by filtration clensed from all dregs) in an earthen broad pan vpon warme ashes: Uapour away the moysture vntill the tincture of the Henbane rootes come to the consistence of Hony, which is very swéet and pleasant. After this, take all these (being beaten to powder) of the séedes of white Poppy one Ounce, of Mummia one scruple, of Cloues and Cinamon, of each 2. Ounces, of Louage roots, Calamus, Arcmaticus, Galingale and Ginger, of each one Ounce, of Castorium, blacke Pepper, Cubebs and Saffron, of each halfe an Ounce, of Ladanum and Beniamin, of each 2.3. Put all these together in a glasse hauing a narrow mouth, which will holde a pottle, and poure in so much good and strong Aqua Vitæ as wil be aboue them foure inches,

of the *Struma*. 47

inches, then with a Corke and a péece of Leather stop it, and let it stand vntill the Aqua Vitæ be of a darke red colour, shaking it thrée times a day in ye glasse: the Aqua Vitæ being full of tincture, let it bee poured off & strayned, and so much againe be poured on, do this til the Aqua Vitæ can draw no colour. Then take all the tinctured Aqua Vitæ, and in Balnea Mariæ in a great glasse body, distill it vntill the tinctures doe come to the consistence of a Syrope: Afterwardes poure them in a broad earthen glased pan, and on warme Ashes by euaporation bring them to the consistence and body of a Pill, which Malax with 2. drams of the oyle of Cloues, let the masse be kept in a cleane glasse.

The Dose is from thrée graines to fiue, to procure sléepe, to aswage the paines of those that are troubled with the Collicke, with the Plurisie, with the Stone, and with the Goute: to stay the Cough, the Fluxe of the Belly, spitting of bloud, and Deflurions of humours, &c. It is said, it were as good for a Chirurgian that followeth the warres, eyther by Sea or Land, to bee without his right hand, as to bee without these remedyes last rehearsed. My selfe haue knowne cured of *Dysenteria*, or the bloudy Flix, and other Fluxes of the belly in a Shippe (being vpon the coaste of Indyes) forty Marriners and Soldiers at one time, and not one of them all perished, by the discréet administration of the said remedyes by seruantes of mine. Within the Citty of London also there be aliue at this present day, which were cured of the Fluxe of the belly, by the forenamed remedyes, when they were supposed of many to be past all recouery, by reason also of the long continuance and their extreame weakenes withall: And here I wish the like good successe vnto others (which I my selfe haue had héereby) that is the onely cause I haue héere made so large mention thereof.

Diuers cured of Dysenteria, or the bloudy Flixe and other Fluxes of the belly.

A most

A most miraculous Cure, healed onely by the Queenes most excellent Maiesty, when neither Phisicke nor Chirurgery could take place or preuaile.

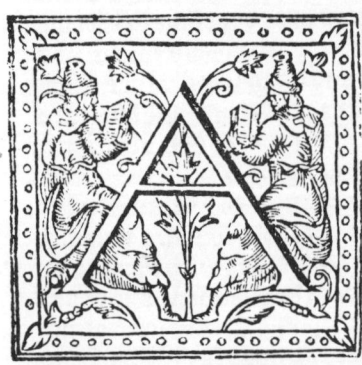

Mongst an infinite nũber (which I haue knowne dayly cured by her Highnes, of the foresaid euill) this cure following is worthy of great admiratiõ: there came into my handes not many yeares past, a certayne Stranger, borne (as he said) in the Land of Gulicke neere vnto Cleaueland. This Stranger had béen in Cure a long time before he came vnto me, with diuers skilfull Chirurgians, both English and Strangers, being then greatly molested and sore troubled with diuers pernitious Cancerous Fistulous Vlcers in certaine places of his body; likewise he had many knotty swellings or abscessions, gathered together vpon heapes in the fore part of his necke, néere vnto the Winde-pipe, and some in the hinder part of the necke: and also amongst the principall and notable vessels, viz. the great Sinewes, Vaines and Arteryes, and therefore could not without great perill and danger be safely taken away, eyther by Launce or Causticke remedies, by reason of their néere knitting together, & were also very vnfit, to be brought to suppuration. The cause was, they were for the most part ingendred of dull and slowe or tough

slymie

of the *Struma*.

slimie matter, for the which I craued now and then the aduyce and counsaile of diuerse learned and expert Phisitians and Chirurgians, onely to preuent and auoide those pernitious daungers that oftentimes doe follow: Howbeit, (in conclusion) notwithstanding all our turmoiling, much care, industry and diligence, with the application of most excellent medicines (very remediable and appropriat for that cure) yet was his griefe rather the worse then better. For looke what way soeuer we tooke with approued medicines, some milde, some vehement, and some stronger (which by naturall reason and common sense, were very good and commendable) yea, and which brought oftentimes all his Ulcers to bee very nære whole: Yet vpon a sodaine (without any iust cause to vs knowne) his sores did putrifye and breake foorth againe, with much loathsome filthinesse, so that I feared his Ulcers would gangrenize, by reason of the concursion and vigour of the vnexpected accidents, so that his disease wearied vs all. In the end, after hee had bæn twelue or thirtæne monethes in my cure, perceiuing we all mist of our expected hope and purpose for the curing of this Infirmity: And likewise himself being ouertyred with extreame paines and griefe, so that oftentimes hee bewailed his owne great misery and wretchednes: for which cause hee went his waies, and came no more vnto mee for any cure: but by the counsaile of some of his owne countrimen and friends, made meanes (vnknowne to me) vnto other of my fellowes the Quænes Maiesties Chirurgians, which are in place of preferment before mæ. Who pitying his miserable estate, vpon a time (amongst many others) he was then presented vnto our most Sacred and renowmed Prince the Quænes most excellent Maiesty, for the cure of the said Euill: which through the gift and power of Almightie God, by her

H   Graces

Graces onely meanes laying of her blessed and happie handes vpon him, shee cured him safely within the space of sixe monthes. Heereby it appeareth it is a more diuine then humane worke, so afterwards vpon a time I did meete with him by chaunce in London, but I did not wel know him, his Colour & complexion was so greatly altered & amended: And being in very comely maner attired, otherwise then before I had seene him, and he tolde me who he was: Then I asked him how he did with his griefe: he answered me, I thank God and the Queene of England, I am by her Maiesty perfectly cured and healed: and after her Grace had touched me, I neuer applyed any Medicine at all, but kept it cleane, with sweet and fresh cleane cloathes, and nowe and then washed the sore with white Wine: and thus all my griefes did consume and waste cleane away. And that I should credit him the more, he shewed mee the Angell of golde which her Maiesty did put about his neck, truely a cure (as I haue said) requireth diuine honour and reuerence: And heere I doe confidently affirme and stedfastly beleeue, that (for the certaine cure of this most miserable Malady) when all Artes and Sciences doe faile, her Highnesse is the onely Day-starre, peerelesse and without comparison: for whose long life, much happines, peace and tranquillity, let vs all (according to our bounden dutyes) continually pray vnto the Almighty God, that he will blesse, keepe and defend her Sacred person, from the malice of all her knowne and vnknowne enemies, so that shee may for euer raigne ouer vs, (if it please the Lord God) euen vnto the ende of the world, still to cure and heale many thousands moe, then euer she hath yet done. Amen.

An

An History and obseruation of a
Gentleman which sent for me, to cure him of the foresaid Euill, but it prooued otherwise.

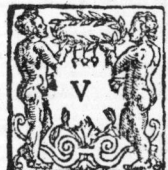

Vpon a time I was sent for to a Gentleman, lying in a Marchantes house at Broken-wharfe in London: after I was brought into his presence, he did forthwith giue me to vnderstand, ỹ he was greatly polluted & molested with much impurity of corrupt & rotten matter, with great exulceration in his throate, being of a filthy and carrionish sauour: also the Almond of his throate was grieuous and painful vnto him, & meruailously swolne: for the which cause (he said) he entertained (a litle before) one D. Simonds, a very learned and Iudiciall Phisitian, who (as he reported) did administer a dyet to him for certaine daies, but it appeared he was smally relieued therby. And further he laide open vnto mee, that of late there was commended vnto him a New-come Stranger, who (vpon report) was supposed to be ỹ onely Phœnix of the world, for his rare and exquisite knowledge in Phisicke and Chirurgery: I answered the Gentleman, that those spæches were so absurd as nothing could be more, for (said I) it is impossible for one mã to haue all knowledge in himself, but it is truely said: One man may know, that which another knoweth not. Well quoth he, I perceiue I haue takẽ a wrong pig by ỹ eare, and so haue brought my hogs to a faire market, & therefore I know not what to say: & I doubt me I shal find a wofull experience, of that he hath practised on me: And therfore said, he I pray you let me haue your good help

It is truely said, giue a man a name to be an early riser though hee lye in bed till noone, it is no great matter.

H 2   in

in curing of me, for preuenting farther danger. Indéede he is more to be esteemed that preuenteth a danger before it doth come, then hee that doth cure it after it is come; Wel said he, the first time he had giuen me a litle Phisicke, hee did very boldly corrosiue mee in two seuerall places of my throate, and yet neuerthelesse I receiued no profit thereby, but hee hath tormented me greatly: So in the end he prayed me to vnbinde his grief, where the corrosiue was applyed, which was directly vpon the outward part of the Amigdales or Kernels of the roote of the tongue, but as good hap was, he being a fat man, the Caustick wrought not too déep: also he shewed mee diuers nodosities, knobs and knottes vpon his shin bones. Then I tolde the Gentleman it was not the Kings Euill: when he heard me speake these words, he was in a wonderfull rage, and did sweare like a mad man. By the way yée shall vnderstand, that this gentlemans vices excéeded his vertues, hee was a man knowne to be as vnconstant & vncertaine as the weather-cock: won with a feather & lost with a straw, to day a friend, to morrow none: at one time he would magnifye his Phisitian and Chirurgian (as it were) aboue the heauens, and for the wagging of a rush, hee would discredit them & dispraise them againe, downe to the pit of hell. But to returne vnto my matter, from whence I haue a litle digressed, forsooth in all poste hast this good Gentleman would néedes haue me ride into the Country to his house (being fifty miles from London) to cure him there: But I tolde him, it was not possible, for that I was dayly to attend vpon the Lord Thomas Earle of Sussex, then being Lord Chamberlaine vnto her Maiesty. In the meane space there came in his Phisitian and Chirurgian whome he reported before to be matchlesse, and without comparison in Phisicke

of the *Struma.*

ficke and Chirurgery: but the cafe is altered, for now he did againe, moſt bitterly reuile him, for miſtaking of his griefe: I muſt nǽds ſay, his Phiſitian was a man of a curteous inclination, and partly after ſpǽches had, he did confeſſe his error and ouer-ſight: yet he ſaid hee had bǽn a profeſſor of this faculty forty yéeres, and indǽd he had the teſtimonies of many great townes and Cityes beyond the Seas, of diuers whome hee had cured of the Kings Euill: To iudge and iudge aright, (as I tolde the Gentleman) hee did nothing of ſet purpoſe to abuſe him, for truely he was learned, though a bad Phiſitian and a worſe Chirurgian. How be it, the worſt I liked in him, was for that he boaſted, and ſaid he was a Chirurgian naturalized, and ſo borne a Chirurgian: truely I tolde him it was a reaſon as naked as my naile: For be it graunted that his Father might bee a good Chirurgian (as him ſelfe reported to vs) what is that to the purpoſe, if his Sonne be found a counterfeit? It is a true ſaying, the beſt Apple will growe to be a Crab, vnleſſe ſome good fruite be grafted on the ſtocke: But indǽde I doe know there bee ſome whoſe Fathers were good Chirurgians, and ſo be their Sonnes likewiſe, but how commeth it to paſſe they bee ſo? Truely the reaſon is, they were like vnto their Fathers, men carefull and painfull in ſtudy, and of long experience. But otherwiſe, for any one to ſuppoſe or dreame, ỹ the Arte commeth to a man by ſucceſſion, becauſe happily his Father was a good Chirurgian, it is a Paradoxicall opinion, very fooliſh, abſurde and fantaſticall: Other the like ſpǽches hee had to this ende and purpoſe, and thus we ended, and ſo I took my leaue, and left them altogether. After I was gone, they fell out with great and vnſéemely wordes: whereupon the Gentleman cauſed his men to ſet his Phiſitian downe in a Chaire, and then with a payre of Taylors ſhǽres,

Where ignorance is clad in learned weede, Small helpe is there to be had in time of neede.

H 3 one

one of his men played Barba tonsoris, and so did Cutte off his faire beard, and shore off the hayre of his head very vnseemely, being a man of his yeeres, and so put him out of doores, without any consideration for his paines and Medicines hee had bestowed vpon him: but what became of him afterward I haue not heard. Then he sent to D. Simonds againe, & tolde him how his new come Phisitiā & Chirur: had abused him & desired him of all friendship to help him presently to some cunning Chirurgian, to cure him forthwith if it were possible, & that with speed: After some talke, the Doctor remembred himselfe, and tolde him he would send him a neighbour of his, one Ma. Story, a Chyrurgian of S. Bartholmewes Hospitall, & a man (said he) wel experienced in his Arte. After he was come home to his house, he did conuerse with his neyghbour M. Story, & tolde him what maner of hasty man the Gent. was: therfore he willed him, saying, before you meddle with him make your bargaine wisely now he is in paine, for hee is but a bad pay-master, and therefore follow this rule. Accipe dum dolet, cum sanus soluere nolet.

As cunning as Master Storye thought to haue been, hee could not get one penny out of his purse, not in sixe daies after hee vndertooke to cure him, vntill Master Story was going away, and said, sir I cannot goe to the market with wordes, but the Gentleman would not heare on that side. Then the Doctor went with Master Story, and tolde the Gentleman: Sir if you ride your horse all day, and giue him no meate at night, and so againe all the next day, you may bee sure you are like to goe a foote the third day. Indeede I remember a pretty saying of one, whose wordes in effect were these: When a Phisitian or a Chyrurgian commeth to a man that lyeth sicke, and is in daunger of death, yet by his iudgement and skill, promiseth with

Gods

of the *Struma*.

Gods helpe, to cure him of his griefes and Maladyes: then the sicke Patient greatly reioyceth, & presently compareth him to a God: But after, being somewhat recouered and perceiueth good amendment, then he doth say, hee is but an Angell, & not a God: Againe, after hee doth walke abroad and falleth to his meate, truely he is then accompted no better then a man: in the end when he happily commeth for his money for the curing of his grieuous sicknes, he now reporteth him to be a deuill, & so shut the doore; Non est inuentus; come when I send for you. To conclude, & now I come againe to speake of Ma. Story, after hee had béen comming and going, twice a day for eyght daies space, hee gaue him certaine money, w̄ a world of faire promises, so far fowrth as he would perfect his Cure at his house in the countrie: But according to the old saying in Latin, Mel in ore verba lactis fel in corda fraus in factis, as by the sequell shall appeare.

At much intreatie hee consented, and went downe to his house in the Country: when hee came vnto the Gentlemans house with him, hee tolde Master Storie saying: I haue a Store-house of diseases and impedimentes in my body, and so I haue not ledde a Saintes life: as hee confessed very strange and far from all good, to this ende (he sayd hee spake it) wherby hee might bee the better instructed to make his cure the more certayne: Then hee tolde the Gentleman hee would be loath to begin a thing when the ende is doubtfull and daungerous, and vnto him before altogether vnknowne: And therefore desired him to send for some skilfull Phisitian or Chirurgian, for further counsaile to his good. Then he did sweare & stare, that he did not bring him downe to expostulate and make Lectures vnto him, but he said he did vnderstand by M.D. Simondes, that he was able to performe greater cures then his was, without the counsel of any
other,

other, and tolde Maſter Story he ſhould not depart aliue out of his houſe, if hee did not perfectly cure him. I truſt (ſayd Maſter Story) you will not (what ſoeuer you ſay) commit ſo foule a fault in your owne houſe, wherby may follow vnto you ſuch diſhonour: Howbeit, Maſter Story was greatly troubled in minde, and ſeeing no remedy, he endeuoured himſelfe with great care and induſtry, to attempt the ſaid Cure, according to the Gentlemans owne requeſt, which was with the Unction: but firſt he prepared and afterwards purged his body, and opened a vaine, and after very diſcreetly hee did adminiſter the Unction at ſeuerall times, vntill hee did ſee and perceiue it had wrought ſufficiently, and to Maſter Stories owne good liking, and ſo meant to haue ceaſed. But this monſter in humanity (contrary to all Arte and reaſon) compelled Maſter Storie to adminiſter the Unction once againe, ſaying his body was ſtrong enough to endure it. Howbeit, within three dayes after, he did begin to ſing a new ſong, for ſtrange and vnexpected accidents immediatly did follow: A great and an inordinate Fluxe of vicious and corrupt humours paſſed out of his mouth, with much acrimony, burning heate and ſharpnes, by reaſon of the putrifaction of his gummes, with an horrible ſtincking ſauour and a Feuer accompanying the ſame: Then he and all his people about him, were in great doubt of his recouery, ſaying to Maſter Story, my griefe (I feare me) will prooue inſanable and deadly. Maſter Story ſaid he hoped not ſo, for you may thanke your ſelf of this extremitie: Then ſecretly (doubting he ſhould dye) he ſent an olde truſtie ſeruant of his to London in all poſte haſte for me, with a Letter ſubſcribed by a wrong name, and by his man 20. Angels. After I had peruſed his letter, and vnderſtood in what a bad caſe he was, I prepared all things neceſſary, and ſo with all expedition ridde
poſt

of the Struma. 57

poaste away with his guide. But when I came into his house where he lay, I did not knowe him, his disease had so altered the naturall shape of his face: at last he reuealed him selfe vnto me, and said, Master Clowes, I haue sent for you, hoping you wil saue my life, I haue béene abused by counterfeit bungling botchers, for one tolde me I had the K. Euill, and an other, I haue the Fr. P. but what soeuer it is, I pray you bend your endeuour and diligence, that with al conuenient spéed I may be brought to my former health, which I know (sayd he) resteth in the skill of a good Chirurgian. After I vnderstood what hee was, I repented mee of my comming, & wisht my selfe at London againe, & his 20. Angels in his belly. To procéede, I tolde him hee was not without danger, & therfore I could not make any warrant of his cure, but the best I could do he should be sure of: then this cankred chuffe looked on me like one that had lately come out of the deuils slaughter-house, & said: if he dyed vnder my cure, there were in his house, that should take accompt of me before I went. Then I tolde him, if he or any of his durst touch or abuse one haire of my head, it would bee déerely answered. But before I procéed any farther, you shal vnderstand, I was informed by one of the Gentlemens men, that M. Story was kept in obscurity (& as it were in a close prison.) So vpō a sodaine, about 10. a clock at night, this Gentle. sent a swash buckler of his own training vp, who was vnto him (as it were) the very light of his eyes, & one that serued him in a nūber of bad matters: He came to M. Story & caused him to rise out of his bed, and bad him prepare to ride towardes London, for hee said he had ordained horses for him selfe, & you M. Story, &c. I will soone bee ready to attend vpon you, said hee, but first (he said) hee would faine haue taken his leaue of the Gent: but this Royster tolde him it was in vaine, his Master had no

Some say, It is not good to speake the truth at all times.

I pleasure

pleasure in the sight of his person: So they took horse, & towards London they did ride, vntill they came into a very great wood farre from any house or towne, and in the midst of the wood bee forced Master Storie to a-light, with many scoffes and scornes, and being very darke, left him to shift for himselfe, where hee wandred vp and downe all the night, with great feare, sorrow and care, till it was day, & then in the end he came into London hye way, and so being ouer-wearyed, rested himselfe for a space, and in the end went to his house in London. After, when this grislie ghost (his man) came home, in the morning hee informed his good Master, how he had dealt with Master Story, whereat (though he being sore and sicklie) yet hee smiled, and greatly reioyced at this bad action: which I did heare, & full wel vnderstood though I said litle, whatsoeuer I thought, but marke hereafter the end of the Master and the man: and now I come againe to my owne procéedings, that is. The morning after Ma. Story was gone, I administred vnto this Gentleman a Glister, made of new Milke, Suger and Oyle of Almonds, which could in no wise haue been lawfully prohibited, by reason of the great restriction and torments of his belly, for hee had not a stoole in fiue dayes before. Now I suppose some vpon a spleane, will obiect against me, and say, that I goe (here and in other places of this booke) beyond my latchet, in the publishing & administring of phisical remedies, vnto my Patients: But I must craue pardon to answere with fauour this obiectió, for be it without offence spoké: I say, where the learned Phisitian is not to be had, be it either by sea or land, far or néer, I wil thé vse al honest & lawful meanes, both in Phisicke & Chi-rurgery, to the vttermost of my knowledge and skill, before I will any way permit ant suffer my Patient to perish for want of all helpe. Notwithstanding, what
  soeuer

of the *Struma*.

soeuer is said and spoken to the contrarie by any malicious aduersary, I assure my selfe, the graue, wise and learned will not take offence at these my sayings, but passe it ouer with modesty & silence. Secondly, though he were weake, by reason of his extreame sweates, paines, and burning heate of his mouth, throate and whole body, for which cause I did let him blood on the Cæphalica vaine, on the right arme, that was, 4. Ounc. of blood in the morning, and 3. Ounces of blood more at foure of the clocke in the after noone the same day. And thus by intermission of time, I took away 7. Oun. of very corrupt and impure blood: this done, I vsed frications, and I set strong cupping glasses vpon his shoulders and hippes, and at sundry times I did administer vnto him certaine comfortable cordials: And then with excellent Gargarismes and Lotions, I brought away many foule and filthye Askers from his mouth and throate: thus within the space of sixe daies, hee did confesse some little ease and amendment, by these inward and outward medicaments. And at the full end of 18 daies after following, I made him perfectly whole, in the meane time hee did cogitate (as it were) and bethought with himselfe, how cunningly he had dealt with his two former Chyrurgians, and did greatly reioyce in this sending them away vnsatisfied. Then I tolde him, it was to Master Storyes great detriment, & hurt vnto his body, and hindrance to his liuing being a poore man: but hee would not heare on that side. Notwithstanding, it is a true saying: It is an ill winde that bloweth no man good; I meane, happy is hee that commeth in the declination and ending of a Cure: and so I let him alone with his humours, sith my reasons was not of force to perswade him: howbeit, in conclusion he vsed me very kindly, & willed me to goe abroad with him, to see his Riuers, wherein were

I 2   many

many goodly Trowtes and other fine fishes, and after shewed me his mighty high woods, and a number of Heronshew-nestes: But truely, I tooke as much pleasure at the sight thereof, as Iacke an Apes doth when he hath a whip at his tayle. After all these sightes, he returned to his house, and by the way he said, Master Clowes, I will holde you no longer with me, but I will send you with my men to London, for I must confesse I haue stayed you longer time then I meant to haue done: and in conclusion, he gaue me 20. pound, and promised mee to rest my assured good friend during his life. But to conclude, I note his vnfortunate end, whereby it presaged he was borne vnder some vnluckie Planet or Crosse day. For within fewe yeeres after, he took occasion to ride abroad, as at many other times he vsed to doe, but in returning home to his owne house, it was said, he entring into a Lane, and attempting to open a great gate, sodainly his horse started aside, and fled away, whereby the Gentleman fell from his horse vnto the ground, and there sodainly brake his owne necke: So his horse ran home, and he being left behinde, the seruants went and sought for him, and found him starke dead, and his necke broke: Thus far of the end of the Master, now to the end of his man, which he appointed to be Master Scoryes guide, the onely Phœnix, whom he déerely loued, but not for his good conditions. Within a yéere after his Ma. came to his vntimely death, (whose end was onely to God foreknown & prefixed) this swaggering fellow did sodainly grow into great misery, & so vpon a time hee came to London, and there I saw him: presently hee craued of mee some reliefe, for hee said, for want of seruice hee was brought into great pouerty: Indéede I must confesse I had small deuotion vnto him, but yet I gaue him some what to be rid of his company: thus he went his waies, saying, he did hope

He liued wickedly & dyed miserably.

it

of the Struma. 61

it would be better or worse with him shortly. Indéed it was reported that not long after, he did consort with a crew of his old companions, & they together immediatly robbed certain Cloathiers of the west country, & being al take, were at y̌ Assises hanged on y̌ gallows at Ailes-bury or there abouts, for the said fact. Thus (friendly Readers) you haue heard (as it were) the tragical histo-ry of the foresaid Gentleman and his man. The cause which hath moued mee to publish the same is, to fore-warne al young practisers of this faculty of Chirurge-ry, being indéed truely called filius Artis, to beware and take héede how they goe, and where and with whome they goe, especially into strange and vnknowne places, and vnto me of such extraordinary & strange qualities, which make but a iest & pastime at the abusing of any man, be he of neuer so much worth, honesty & skil in his profession.

A fit Pulpit for such a Prophet.

An obseruation for the Cure
of Struma, performed by me vpon a woman dwelling in the County of Essex. 1602.

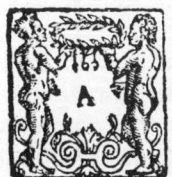
Mongst others that I haue cured this present yéere Anno 1602. there repay-red vnto me, a woman being about the age of thirtye yéeres, dwelling in the County of Essex, thrée miles from my now dwelling house at Plasto, in the parish of Westham, within the said County: which woman was a long time molested and troubled with certaine Carnosityes and hard Strumous swellinges vnder her Chinne, some moueable and some vnmoue-able: the which woman I did take in cure, for the said infirmity, and after spéeches had, I perswaded her

that

that shee would permit mee to take her Strumous swellings away by Incision, but it fell out shee shewed her selfe faint-hearted, and so vnwilling to suffer that action by Incision. Notwithstanding, shee hauing an ardent desire and affection to bee cured by mee, was very willing to indure and abide the force and painfull working of the Causticke, which was performed as followeth.

The incredible operation of this simple Causticke now following is aboue beliefe, being indéed made but onely of the powder of new quick burnt Lime-stones, as they come out of the Kyll, and of Sope well mixed together, An.q.s. Héere some peraduenture wil say, it is a great vanity in mée, to commend a remedie which is well knowne already, (it will doe that it is prescribed for) but I will leaue to answere such obiections, and will procéede with matter of more importance, that is to wit: After I had well defended the partes about, then I applyed vpon these swellinges, the aforesaid Causticke, which she reasonable well endured, for the space of thrée houres: and then I remooued it, and in place thereof I applyed other medicaments, onely to mollifye and loose the Askers, which was made by the said Causticke, and also I gaue with her (of the same remedy) home to her house, to dresse her selfe with all: where shee remained for the space of fiue daies, in the end yée shall note, she returned againe to me, being very faint, pale and ill coloured, thereat I much maruailed, to sée so sodaine an alteration: then I demaunded the reason of her, shee answered and said it was by reason of the bad sent and ill sauours of the Askers, and of the filthy corrupt matter, which did run from the foresaid Cauterized Strumous swellings, that greatly offended her stomacke, and by reason of the sensibilitie of the grieued partes, which were sharpe, mordant and byting,

byting, and that was after the Akers were remooued: and further, she confessed in the end, that she was quick with childe, which troubled her greatly, all which causes being considered, I very much feared an vntimely birth, but I tolde her she was much too blame, that she did not acquaint me therewith, before I tooke her in cure. Howbeit, God did so open my knowledge and vnderstanding, that all thinges fell happily out, better then we looked for. So after, I appointed her to bee drest twise a day with conuenient remedies, and then by the vse of some metalline instruments, onely to apprehend and to pull out part of the foresaid Strumous swellings. So, according as I haue said before, those which are Masters and Professors, chosen to performe the like operation, ought indéede to haue a Lyons heart, a Ladies hand, and a Haukes eye, for that it is a worke of no smal importance. Then by the applycation of these two noble compositions, being irrepromugable and most iudicially penned, and of great truth and probability in this cure, that is Vnguentũ Apostolorũ mesux, & Vnguentum Ægiptiacum, with other worthy Agglutinatiues and drying medicaments, often times before named, and thus she was perfectly cured within the space of 10. wéeks. Friendly Reader, ỹ cause chiefly which hath moued mee to publish this obseruation amongst therest, is partly (as I haue before said) to render some fruites of my labours, studies and time spent, which as it may héere appeare, is no afternoone mans worke, as some rake-shames & belly Gods haue falsly and slaunderously so reported: but the troth is I haue carefully laboured héere, also to admonish euery yonng practiser of Chirurgery, which is rightly called filius Artis, that hee in no wise attempt thē like cure, vpon any woman with childe, without some sage aduise: for great was the troubles and daungers

that

that was like to haue followed, but happily were they preuented through the helpe of Almighty God, &c. Now heere I will forbeare any further to discourse herein, but I will set downe certaine Prescriptions worthy of obseruing, which I haue gathered out of Plinie, (a most worthy writer) for the cure of the fore named Euill, the which I wil heere set downe word for word, as followeth.

The cure of the King or Queenes Euill, after Plinius Secundus description.

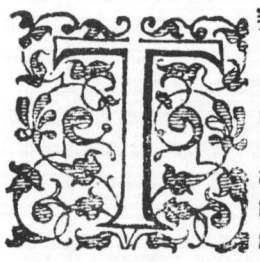

The bloud of a Weisell is good for the Wennes called the King or Queenes Euill, when they be exulcerate and doe run: so is the Weysell it selfe sod in Wine, and applyed. Prouided alwaies, that they run not by the occasion of any launcing or Incision, made by the Chirurgians hand: and it is commonly said, that to eate the flesh of a Weisell is as effectuall for the cure: so are the Ashes of a Wetzell calcined vpon the fire made of Wine twigs, if they be incorporated with Hogs grease. Item, take a groene Lyzard and binde it to the fore, but (after thirtie daies) you must doe so with another, and this wil heale them. Some make no more a doe, but in a little boxe of siluer, keepe the heart of a Weisell, and weare it about them. If a Woman or a Maide bee troubled with the Kings or Queenes Euill, it were good to make a Plaister or Linament of old shell Snailes, and
let

of the *Struma*.

let them be ſtamped ſhelles and all (eſpecially ſuch as be ſticking to the rootes of ſhrubbes or buſhes. The Aſhes of a Serpent Aſpis calcyned are likewiſe very good for this diſeaſe, if they be incorporated with Buls Tallow, and ſo applyed. Some vſe Snakes greaſe and Oyle together: alſo a Linament made of the aſhes of Snakes burnt, tempered with Oyle and Waxe. Moreouer, it is thought that the middle part of a Snake (after the head and tayle bee both cut away) is very wholeſome meate for thoſe that haue the Kinges Euill: or to drinke the Aſhes, being in the same maner prepared, burnt in a new Earthen pot neuer occupyed. Marry, if the ſaid Snakes chaunce to be killed betwéene two Cart trackes where the whéele went, the Medicine will worke much more effectuall. Some giue counſell to apply vnto the affected place Crickets digged out of the earth, with the moulde and all that commeth vp: alſo to apply Pigeons dung, onely without any thing elſe, or at the moſt tempered with Barly meale, or Ote-meale in Vineger: likewiſe, to make a Linament of Mouldwarpes aſhes, incorporate with Vony. Some there be that take the Liuer of a Moule cruſhed and bruiſed betwéene their hands, working it to a Linament, and lay the ſame to the ſore, and there let it dry vpon the place, and waſh it not in thrée dayes. And they affirme that the foote of a Moulde is a ſinguler good remedy for this diſeaſe: others catch ſome of them, and cut off their heads, ſtampe them with the moulde that they haue wrought and caſt vp aboue ground, and reduce them into certayne trocheſces, which kéepe in a boxe or potte of Tinne, and vſe them by way of applycation, to all Tumours and Impoſtumes, which the Grǽkes call Apoſthemata, and eſpeciallie thoſe that ryſe in the Necke: but then they forbid the Patient to eate Porke, or any Swine,

K   during

during the Cure. Moreouer, there is a kinde of earth-Béetles, called Tauri or bulles, which name they took of the little Hornets that they carry, for otherwise in colour they resemble Tickes, some terme them Pediculos terrarum or earth Lice: these worke also vnder the ground like Wantes, and cast vp moulde which serueth in a Linament for the Kings Euill, and such like swellings: also for the Goute in the feete, but it must not be washed off in thrée dayes space. Howbeit, this is to be noted, that the medicine must be renewed euery yéere, for the same moulde will continue no longer in vertue then one yéere: In some, there be attributed vnto Béetles, all those medicinall properties which I haue assigned vnto Crickets called Grillj. Moreouer, some there be, who vse (in maner and cases aforesaid) the moulde which Antes doe cast vp. Others (for the Kinges Euill) take vp as many Maddes or Earth-wormes in number, as there be Wennes gathered and knotted together, and binde the same fast vnto them, letting them dry vpon the place, and they are perswaded that the same Wennes will dry and consume away together with them. There be againe, who doe get a Viper, about the rising of the Dog-starre, cutting off the head and tayle, (as I said before of the Snakes) and the middle part betweene they burne: the Ashes that come thereof, they giue afterwards to drinke for thrée wéekes together, euery day as much as may be comprehended and taken vp at thrée fingers endes, and thus they cure the Kings Euill. Moreouer, there bee some which hang a Viper by a Linnen thréed, fast tyed somewhat vnder the head, so long till shee be strangled and dead, and with that thréed binde the Wennes or Kings Euill aforesaid, promising vnto the Patient assured remedye thereby. They vse also the Solues called Multipedæ, & incorporate the same with a fourth
part

part in proportion of them, of true Turpentine: and they be of that opinion, that this Oyntement or Salue is sufficient to cure any Impostumes whatsoeuer. Ætius also sayth, if a man should eate a Viper, it is a most notable thing: whose authority others also haue followed in administring vnto Strumous persons Trochiscos Viperinos, or the Pilles of Vipers, with good & happy successe. Also it was said, it was the experience in times past of countrymen, that if any had eaten a Snake, hee should bee deliuered from Struma. Thus much touching Pliny his manner and order which hee hath published, for the Curing the Kings or Quænes Euill.

The conclusion.

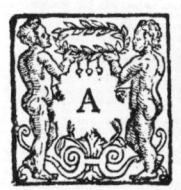

And thus (friendly Reader) it were a great argument of folly & shameles impudency in me, worthy to be laughed at, once to think that I could héer any way instruct the learned Phisitiã or Chirurgian, in the Cure of the Kinges or Quænes Euill, before named. I am not so full of childish toyes: but if I were, I doe full well know they might by their prouident wisedomes and learning easily circumuent mee, though I doe confesse, I am not altogether insufficient to performe this enterprize I haue héere set downe and taken in hand. The onely cause why I haue done it, is (as I haue before said) for the benefit of all young Students of Chirurgery, who haue a long time expected the comming foorth and the publishing of this Booke: whose honest zeale and affection towards me, hath induced mee the rather to set foorth the same. But before I would attempt it without good aduise, I did first intreate diuers

Phisitians and Chirurgians (men of a singuler perceiuerance, in perusing and examining the same) of whom I haue had a fauourable acceptation: And this I did of purpose, least some might (otherwise) lay stumbling blocks in my way, onely to impeach these my painfull labors & trauels. And so I do make a final end, acknowledging as I did in ye beginning, That the gift of healing, is the gift of God: howbeit, I doe not heere presume, or once take vpon me to enter into the high cure of the said Euill vsually called Schrophula, in such wise as God hath giuen diuine & peculiar giftes vnto Princes: but my full intent hath alwaies been onely to direct the true path-way of Artificial gifts (wch God of his great goodnes giueth to men of Arte) knowledge & skil in Phisick & Chirurgery, wch is performed & done by the applicatiõ of interiall & exteriall medicamentes, appropriate & approued profitable therfore. For it is a true saying: God hath created medicines of the earth, for the reliefe & comfort of man; and it is said: He that is wise wil not refuse it. And thus last of all, I thought it not impertinent, heere to diuert & digresse frõ the matter, & wholy attribute all diuine honor & reuerence, for the great cure of the forenamed Euill, (by Gods gratious good gifts) vnto our most prouidẽt, wise & vertuous Princesse, the Queenes most Royall Maiesty: For whom let vs all pray, that the Lord God Almighty & eternal Sauiour wil send her Highnes still long and long to raigne ouer vs, to our great ioy, happines & comfort, so that she may liue long, and many happy yeeres & daies, to hold vp the Scepter of this Kingdome, in Christ Iesus. Amen.

The Lord of Hoastes, preserue these coastes,
 Our gratious Queene defend:
 And graunt her peace may still increase,
  Vntill this world shall end.

FINIS.

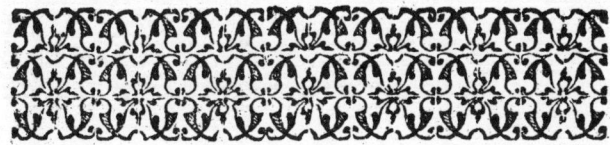

FRiendly Reader, I hope you shal not think your time & trauel mispent, if you will be pleased to vouchsafe, with diligent regard, the carefull reading of this small Treatise: wherein it may so fall out, that some blemishes or ouer-slips hath passed, notwithstanding, all the watchfull eyes and great paines and care hath been taken to the contrarie. For the which, if any such faultes happen to bee, then I desire thee (curteous and friendly Reader) to censure it with fauour, & eyther with your pen amend what is amisse; or otherwise, returne me a friendly admonition, which at the next impression shall willingly be amended, sith at this time the number is not many, which I haue caused to be Printed. Then as for the enuious, idle & ignorant Momus, (of whome I know I shall be priuily pinched) of such bad persons I refuse and disdaine to be censured, and iudged by: And thus I leaue thee (friendly Reader) in the Lord Iesus.

   From my now dwelling house at Plasto, in the
    Parish of Westham, in the Coun-
      ty of Essex.

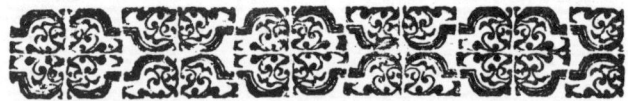

This Booke vvas ex=
amined, seene & allowed to be
Printed, according to order appointed:
And are now to bee solde at Master Lay-
bournes, a Barber Chirurgian dwelling
vpon Saint Mary Hill, neere
Billings-gate.

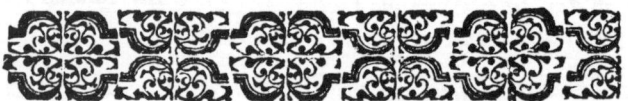

R
128.7
C63
1602a

OCT 5 1971